Chronic Candidiasis—
The Yeast Syndrome

Other Books
by Michael T. Murray

Encyclopedia of Natural Medicine

Encyclopedia of Nutritional Supplements

Natural Alternatives to Over-the-Counter and Prescription Drugs

The Healing Power of Herbs

The Healing Power of Foods

From the GETTING WELL NATURALLY SERIES
 Chronic Fatigue Syndrome
 Menopause
 Male Sexual Vitality
 Arthritis
 Diabetes and Hypoglycemia
 Stress, Anxiety, and Insomnia
 Premenstrual Syndrome
 Stomach Ailments and Digestive Disturbances
 Heart Disease and High Blood Pressure

Natural Alternatives for Weight Loss

Natural Alternatives to Prozac

GETTING WELL NATURALLY SERIES

Chronic Candidiasis— The Yeast Syndrome

Michael T. Murray, N.D.

PRIMA HEALTH
A Division of Prima Publishing

PRIMA HEALTH and its colophon are trademarks of Prima Communications, Inc.

Warning—Disclaimer
Prima Publishing has designed this book to provide information in regard to the subject matter covered. It is sold with the understanding that the publisher and the author are not liable for the misconception or misuse of information provided. Every effort has been made to make this book as complete and as accurate as possible. The purpose of this book is to educate. The author and Prima Publishing shall have neither liability nor responsibility to any person or entity with respect to any loss, damage, or injury caused or alleged to be caused directly or indirectly by the information contained in this book. The information presented herein is in no way intended as a substitute for medical counseling.

Library of Congress Cataloging-in-Publication Data

Murray, Michael T.
    Chronic candidiasis—the yeast syndrome : how you can benefit from diet, vitamins, minerals, herbs, exercise, and other natural methods / Michael T. Murray.
      p.   cm.
    Includes bibiliographical references and index.
    ISBN 0-7615-0821-X
    1. Candidiasis—Alternative treatment.   2. Naturopathy.
  I. Title.
RC123.C3M87   1997
616.9'69—dc21   97-13549
                                                       CIP

99 00 01 HH 10 9 8 7 6 5 4 3
Printed in the United States of America

All products mentioned in this book are trademarks of their respective companies.

How to Order
Single copies may be ordered from Prima Publishing, P.O. Box 1260BK, Rocklin, CA 95677; telephone (916) 632-4400. Quantity discounts are also available. On your letterhead, include information concerning the intended use of the books and the number of books you wish to purchase.

Visit us online at http://www.primahealth.com

About the Author

Michael T. Murray, N.D., is widely regarded as one of the world's leading authorities on natural medicine. He is a graduate, faculty member, and member of the Board of Trustees of Bastyr University in Seattle, Washington. In addition to maintaining a private medical practice, Dr. Murray is an accomplished writer, educator, and lecturer. He is the medical editor of *The American Journal of Natural Medicine.*

Dr. Murray serves on several editorial boards and advisory panels. As a consultant to the health food industry, Dr. Murray has been instrumental in bringing many effective natural products to America, including: ginkgo biloba extract, glucosamine sulfate, silymarin, enteric-coated peppermint oil, bilberry extract, DGL (deglycyrrhizinated licorice), saw palmetto berry extract, and the first thermogenic formula for weight loss.

For the past ten years, Dr. Murray has been compiling a massive database of original scientific studies from the medical literature. He has collected over 50,000 articles from the scientific literature that provide strong evidence of the effectiveness of diet, vitamins, minerals, glandular extracts, herbs, and other natural measures in the maintenance of health and the treatment of disease. It is from this constantly expanding database that Dr. Murray provides the answers on health and healing. According to Dr. Murray:

> *One of the great myths about natural medicines is that they are not scientific. The fact of the matter is that for most common illnesses there is greater support in the medical literature for a natural approach than there is for drugs or surgery.*

Unfortunately for many people, they are never aware of the natural approach that can put them on the road to lifelong health. Michael Murray has dedicated his life to educating physicians, patients, and the general public on the tremendous healing power of nature. In addition to his books, Dr. Murray has written thousands of articles, appeared on hundreds of radio and TV programs, and lectured live to over 200,000 people, nationwide.

Contents

Before You Read On   x

1 An Overview of Chronic Candidiasis
(the Yeast Syndrome)   1

The Yeast Syndrome   1
What Causes Chronic Candidiasis?   2
A Vicious Cycle   2
The Candida Questionnaire   3
Diagnosis of the Yeast Syndrome   8
The Comprehensive Stool and Digestive Analysis   10
Measuring Antibody or Antigen Levels   12
Syndromes Related to the Yeast Syndrome   12
Final Comments   16

2 Antibiotics and the Yeast Syndrome   17

Dependence Upon Antibiotics   18
Alternatives to Antibiotics   19
Bladder Infections   19
Antibiotics and Upper Respiratory Tract Infections   26
Treating Upper Respiratory Infections Naturally   27
Acne   29
Final Comments   32

3 Enhancing Digestive Secretions   35

The Pancreas   38
Final Comments   41

4 Dietary Factors   43

Sugar and the Yeast Syndrome   43
Milk and Dairy Products   45
Mold- and Yeast-Containing Foods   45
Food Allergies   45
Signs and Symptoms of Food Allergies   46
Immune-System Disorders and Food Allergies   51
Other Factors Triggering Food Allergies   52
Diagnosis of Food Allergy   54
Dealing with Food Allergies   57
The Candida Control Diet   63
Final Comments   74

5 Nutritional Supplementation   75

Taking a High-Quality Multiple Vitamin
   and Mineral Supplement   75
Taking Extra Antioxidants   77
Taking One Tablespoon of Flaxseed Oil Daily   80
Final Comments   81

6 Enhancing Immunity   83

What Is the Immune System?   83
Immune Function and Chronic Candidiasis   88
Restoring Proper Immune Function   89
The Influence of Mood and Attitude
   on Immune Function   90
The Influence of Lifestyle on Immune Function   93
Diet and Immune Function   94
Poor Diet Resulting in Nutrient Deficiency   94
Enhancing Thymus Gland Activity   96
Plant-Based Medicines   98
Final Comments   99

7 Promoting Detoxification 101

The Importance of the Liver   101
The Liver and Immune Function   102
Damage to the Liver and Chronic Candidiasis   103
Supporting the Liver   103
Supporting Detoxification by Promoting Elimination   111
Final Comments   112

8 Probiotics 113

Historical Perspective   113
Available Forms of Probiotics   114
Prinicple Uses of Probiotics   116
Promoting a Healthy Intestinal Environment   116
Post-Antibiotic Therapy   118
Fructo-Oligosaccharides   120
Final Comments   120

9 Natural and Prescription Anti-Yeast Agents 123

Natural Anti-Yeast Agents   124
Prescription Anti-Yeast Therapies   127
Final Comments   129

10 Special Concerns for Women: Vaginal Yeast Infections, Vulvodynia, and Premenstrual Syndrome 131

Vaginal Yeast Infections   131
Vulvodynia   136
Premenstrual Syndrome   142
Final Comments   145

11 Putting It All Together 147

References   151

Index   167

Before You Read On

This book was written to empower you regarding your health care decisions; it is not designed to replace appropriate medical care. With that in mind, here are some important recommendations:

- Do not self-diagnose. Proper medical care is critical to good health. If you have symptoms suggestive of an illness, please consult a physician—preferably a naturopath, holistic physician or osteopath, chiropractor, or other natural health care specialist.

- If you are currently on a prescription medication, you absolutely must consult your doctor before discontinuing it. Furthermore, you must make your physician aware of all the nutritional supplements you are currently taking and why.

- If you wish to try a nutritional supplement as a therapeutic measure, discuss it with your physician. Since he or she is most likely unaware of the natural alternatives available, you may need to do some educating. Bring this book along with you to the doctor's office. The natural alternatives being recommended are based on published studies in medical journals. Key references are provided if your physician wants additional information.

- Remember, although many nutritional alternatives, such as nutritional supplements and plant-based medicines, are effective on their own, they work even better if they are part of a comprehensive natural treatment plan that focuses on diet and lifestyle.

Acknowledgments

The major blessings in my life are my family and friends. My love for them truly makes life worth living.

Special appreciation to my wife, Gina, for being the answer to so many of my dreams; to my parents, Cliff and Patty Murray, and my grandmother, Pauline Shier, for a strong foundation and a lifetime of good memories; to Bob and Kathy Bunton for their love and acceptance; to Ben Dominitz and everyone at Prima for their commitment and support of my work; to Terry Lemerond and everyone at Enzymatic Therapy for all of their friendship and support over the years; and to Joseph Pizzorno and the students and faculty at Bastyr College who have given me encouragement and support. And finally, I am eternally grateful to all the researchers, physicians, and scientists who over the years have sought to better understand the use of natural medicines. Without their work, this series would not exist, and medical progress would halt.

Michael T. Murray, N.D.

1

An Overview of Chronic Candidiasis (the Yeast Syndrome)

An overgrowth in the gastrointestinal tract of the usually benign yeast *Candida albicans* has recently been recognized as a complex medical syndrome known as *chronic candidiasis* or the *yeast syndrome*.[1,2] Specifically, the overgrowth of candida is believed to cause a wide variety of symptoms in virtually every system of the body, with the gastrointestinal, genitourinary, endocrine, nervous, and immune systems being the most susceptible.[3]

Although chronic candidiasis has been clinically defined for a long time, it was not until Dr. Orion Truss wrote *The Missing Diagnosis* and Dr. William Crook wrote *The Yeast Connection* that the public and many physicians became aware of the magnitude of the problem.[1,2]

The Yeast Syndrome

Normally *Candida albicans* lives harmoniously in the human body, in the inner warm creases and crevices of the digestive tract (and the vaginal tract in women). However, when this yeast overgrows, immune-system mechanisms are depleted, or the normal lining of the intestinal tract is damaged, the body can absorb yeast cells, particles of yeast cells, and various toxins.[3] As a result, bodily processes may be significantly disrupted, resulting in the development of the yeast syndrome.

This syndrome is characterized by "feeling sick all over." Fatigue, allergies, immune-system malfunction, depression, chemical sensitivities, and digestive disturbances are just some of the symptoms patients with the yeast syndrome may experience.[3]

The typical patient with the yeast syndrome is female (see Table 1.1). Women are eight times more likely to experience the yeast syndrome than men due to the effects of estrogen, birth control pills, and the higher number of antibiotics prescribed for women.[4]

What Causes Chronic Candidiasis?

Chronic candidiasis is a classic example of a *multifactorial* condition. This term means that many factors contribute to the overgrowth of *Candida albicans* (see Table 1.2). Therefore, the most effective treatment involves addressing and correcting the factors that predispose someone toward candida overgrowth and not simply killing the yeast with anti-fungal agents, whether synthetic or natural.

A Vicious Cycle

In normal situations, the body keeps *Candida albicans* in check. But, in the presence of a predisposing factor, the yeast can overgrow and produce a vicious cycle (illustrated by Figure 1.1), which exists in many people with chronic candidiasis and highlights the importance of a comprehensive approach to the problem.

Table 1.1 Typical Chronic Candidiasis Patient Profile

Sex: female	*Immune system complaints:*
Age: 15 to 50	Allergies
	Chemical sensitivities
General symptoms:	Low immune function
Chronic fatigue	*Past history:*
Loss of energy	Chronic vaginal yeast infections
General malaise	Chronic antibiotic use for infec-
Decreased libido	tions or acne
Gastrointestinal symptoms:	Oral birth control usage
Thrush	Oral steroid hormone usage
Bloating, gas	*Associated conditions:*
Intestinal cramps	Premenstrual syndrome
Rectal itching	Sensitivity to foods, chemicals,
Altered bowel function	and other allergens
Genitourinary system complaints:	Endocrine disturbances
Vaginal yeast infection	Psoriasis
Frequent bladder infections	Irritable bowel syndrome
Endocrine system complaints:	*Other:*
Primarily menstrual complaints	Craving for foods rich in carbohy-
Nervous system complaints:	drates or yeast
Depression	
Irritability	
Inability to concentrate	

Table 1.2 Predisposing Factors to Candida Overgrowth

Decreased digestive secretions	Impaired liver function
Dietary factors	Underlying disease states, such as
Impaired immunity	AIDS, immune system disor-
Nutrient deficiency	ders, cancer
Drugs (particularly antibiotics,	Altered bowel flora
birth control pills, and syn-	
thetic estrogen)	

The Candida Questionnaire

One of the most useful screening methods for determining the likelihood of yeast-related illness is a comprehensive questionnaire. The questionnaire that I use is on page 5.

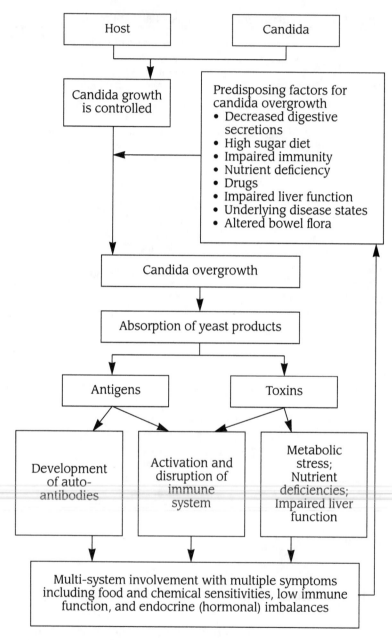

Figure 1.1   The Candida Cycle

Candida Questionnaire

	Point Score

History

1. Have you taken tetracycline or other antibiotics for acne for one month or longer? — 25

2. Have you, at any time in your life, taken other broad-spectrum antibiotics for respiratory, urinary, or other infections for two months or longer, or in short courses four or more times in a one-year period? — 20

3. Have you ever taken a broad-spectrum antibiotic (even a single course)? — 6

4. Have you, at any time in your life, been bothered by persistent prostatitis, vaginitis, or other problems affecting your reproductive organs? — 25

5. Have you been pregnant . . .
   One time? — 3
   Two or more times? — 5

6. Have you taken birth control pills . . .
   For six months to two years? — 8
   For more than two years? — 15

7. Have you taken prednisone or other cortisone-type drugs . . .
   For two weeks or less? — 6
   For more than two weeks? — 15

8. Does exposure to perfumes, insecticides, fabric shop odors, and other chemicals provoke . . .
   Mild symptoms? — 5
   Moderate to severe symptoms? — 20

9. Are your symptoms worse on damp, muggy days or in moldy places? — 20

10. Have you had athlete's foot, ringworm, "jock itch," or other chronic infections of the skin or nails?
    Mild to moderate? — 10
    Severe or persistent? — 20

11. Do you crave sugar? — 10

12. Do you crave breads? — 10

Continued

Candida Questionnaire *(continued)*

13. Do you crave alcoholic beverages?	10
14. Does tobacco smoke *really* bother you?	10

Total Score of This Section _____

Major Symptoms

For each of your symptoms, enter the appropriate figure in the Point Score column.

Score column:

If a symptom is occasional or mild, score 3 points
If a symptom is frequent and/or moderately severe,
   score 6 points
If a symptom is severe and/or disabling, score 9 points

POINT SCORE

1. Fatigue or lethargy	_____
2. Feeling of being "drained"	_____
3. Poor memory	_____
4. Feeling "spacey" or "unreal"	_____
5. Depression	_____
6. Numbness, burning, or tingling	_____
7. Muscle aches	_____
8. Muscle weakness or paralysis	_____
9. Pain and/or swelling in joints	_____
10. Abdominal pain	_____
11. Constipation	_____
12. Diarrhea	_____
13. Bloating	_____
14. Persistent vaginal itch	_____
15. Persistent vaginal burning	_____
16. Prostatitis	_____
17. Impotence	_____
18. Loss of sexual desire	_____
19. Endometriosis	_____
20. Cramps and/or other menstrual irregularities	_____
21. Premenstrual tension	_____

Candida Questionnaire *(continued)*

22. Spots in front of eyes	_____
23. Erratic vision	_____
Total Score of This Section	_____

Other Symptoms

For each of your symptoms, enter the appropriate figure in the Point Score column.

Score column:

If a symptom is occasional or mild, score 1 point
If a symptom is frequent and/or moderately severe,
   score 2 points
If a symptom is severe and/or disabling, score 3 points

POINT SCORE

1. Drowsiness	_____
2. Irritability	_____
3. Incoordination	_____
4. Inability to concentrate	_____
5. Frequent mood swings	_____
6. Headache	_____
7. Dizziness/loss of balance	_____
8. Pressure above ears, feeling of head swelling and tingling	_____
9. Itching	_____
10. Other rashes	_____
11. Heartburn	_____
12. Indigestion	_____
13. Belching and intestinal gas	_____
14. Mucus in stools	_____
15. Hemorrhoids	_____
16. Dry mouth	_____
17. Rash or blisters in mouth	_____
18. Bad breath	_____
19. Joint swelling or arthritis	_____
20. Nasal congestion or discharge	_____
21. Postnasal drip	_____

Continued

Candida Questionnaire *(continued)*

22. Nasal itching   _____
23. Sore or dry throat   _____
24. Cough   _____
25. Pain or tightness in chest   _____
26. Wheezing or shortness of breath   _____
27. Urinary urgency or frequency   _____
28. Burning on urination   _____
29. Failing vision   _____
30. Burning or tearing of eyes   _____
31. Recurrent infections or fluid in ears _____
32. Ear pain or deafness   _____

   Total Score of This Section   _____

   Total Score of All Three Sections   _____

Interpretation

	Women	Men
Yeast-connected health problems are almost certainly present	>180	>140
Yeast-connected health problems are probably present	120–180	90–140
Yeast-connected health problems are possibly present	60–119	40–89
Yeast-connected health problems are less likely present	<60	<40

Adapted from Crook, W. G., *The Yeast Connection,* 2nd ed., Professional Books, Jackson, TN, 1984.

Diagnosis of the Yeast Syndrome

Although using the candida questionnaire can help, the best method for diagnosing chronic candidiasis is a clinical evaluation by a physician knowledgeable about yeast-related illness. More than likely the manner in which the doctor will diagnose the yeast syndrome will be based on a detailed medical history and patient questionnaire. The doctor may also employ laboratory techniques such as stool cultures for candida and measurement of antibody levels to candida or candida antigens in the blood. However, while these laboratory exams are useful diagnostic aids, they should only be used to confirm the diagnosis. In other words, the diagnosis is best made by a thorough evaluation of the patient's history and clinical picture.

Unfortunately physicians knowledgeable about yeast-related illness are not as plentiful as they should be. The conventional medical community has been slow to recognize the role that chronic candida overgrowth plays in health. Nonetheless knowledgeable doctors are out there. To find a physician in your area, contact one (or all) of these professional organizations:

The American Association of Naturopathic Physicians
P.O. Box 20386
Seattle, WA 98102
206-323-7610

The American Academy of Environmental Medicine
4510 West Eighty-ninth Street
Prairie Village, KS 66207
913-642-6062

The American Holistic Medical Association
4101 Lake Boone Trail, Suite 201
Raleigh, NC 26707
919-787-5146

American College of Advancement in Medicine
(ACAM)
23121 Verdugo Drive, Suite 204
Laguna Hills, CA, 92653
1-800-532-3688 (outside California) or
1-800-435-6199 (inside California)

The Comprehensive Stool and Digestive Analysis

Rather than simply culture a stool sample for the presence of *Candida albicans,* I prefer to use the comprehensive digestive stool analysis (CDSA)—a battery of integrated diagnostic laboratory tests that evaluate digestion, intestinal function, intestinal environment, and absorption by carefully examining the stool.[5] It is a very useful tool for determining which digestive disturbances are the likely underlying factors responsible for candida overgrowth. In addition, the CDSA may discover that the symptoms are not related to candida overgrowth but rather to other digestive ailments such as small intestinal bacterial overgrowth and the "leaky gut" syndrome (both are discussed below).

Laboratories that I am familiar with which provide the CDSA are:

Great Smokies Diagnostic Laboratory (1-800-522-4762)

National BioTech Laboratory (1-800-846-6285)

Diagnos-Techs (1-800-87-TESTS)

Meridian Valley Clinical Laboratory (1-206-859-8700)

The CDSA performed by these laboratories provides information that is useful in leading to the correct diagnosis of causes and the development of appropriate treatment. Many physicians consider it a "foundation" screening test that consistently provides valuable clinical information. Proper digestion is a requirement for optimum health and incomplete or disordered digestion can be a major contributor to the development of many diseases, including the yeast syndrome. Determining digestive function and assessing the intestinal environment through the CDSA can provide valuable information as to the cause of the disturbance. This information can then be used to achieve

Table 1.3   Components of the CDSA

Digestion	Colonic Environment
Triglycerides	Beneficial bacteria
Chymotrypsin	Lactobacillus
Meat fibers	Bifidobacteria
Vegetable fibers	E. Coli
Valerate, iso-Butyrate	Pathogenic bacteria
Absorption	Mycology
	Metabolic Markers
Long-chain fatty acids	pH
Cholesterol	Short-chain fatty acid distribution
Total fecal fat	Butyrate
Total short-chain fatty acids	Beta-Glucuronidase
	Immunology
	Fecal secretory IgA
	Macroscopic
	Fecal color
	Mucus
	Occult blood

improved digestion and a more optimal intestinal environment, which prevents the overgrowth of *Candida albicans.*

The test involves following a special diet for at least two days. Each lab has slightly different recommendations: Basically the goal is to eat a variety of foods and avoid laxatives, iron supplements, vitamin C, multivitamin formulas, and digestive enzymes because they may interfere with test results. Table 1.3 lists the individual components that are typically analyzed.

The Value of the CDSA

The CDSA offers valuable information as to the status of the intestinal environment. In addition to determining the presence of *Candida albicans,* the test also provides insight into what factors may be responsible for promoting its overgrowth. Several labs (most notably Great Smokies)

provide sensitivity studies to determine which agents, including natural compounds, can be used to kill candida.

Measuring Antibody or Antigen Levels

Another laboratory method that can confirm the presence of candida overgrowth is measuring the level of antibodies to candida or the level of candida antigens in the blood.[3,6] I rarely order these tests, however, because the results typically only confirm what the patient's history, physical exam, and CDSA reveal. Hence, the test does not change the course of action. Nonetheless, some patients and physicians may desire confirmation that *Candida albicans* is a responsible factor in the patient's health equation. In that situation, these blood studies can be quite helpful and can also be used as way of monitoring therapy. These tests are performed by only a small number of laboratories:

Antibody Assay Laboratory (1-800-522-2611)

Immunodiagnostic Lab (510-635-4545)

National BioTech Laboratory (1-800-846-6285)

Diagnos-Techs (1-800-87-TESTS)

Syndromes Related to the Yeast Syndrome

Eventually the term the *yeast syndrome* will likely be replaced by a more comprehensive term that will include small intestinal bacterial overgrowth and the leaky gut syndrome. Both of these conditions are often associated with *Candida albicans* overgrowth and may produce identical symptoms to the yeast syndrome.

Small Intestinal Bacterial Overgrowth

An overgrowth of bacteria in the small intestine can lead to symptoms identical to the yeast syndrome. The upper portion of the human small intestine is designed to be relatively free of bacteria. The reason is simple—when bacteria are present in significant concentrations in the small intestine they compete with their host (the human body) for nutrition. When bacteria (or yeast) get to the food first, problems can occur. The organisms can ferment the carbohydrates and produce excessive gas, bloating, and abdominal distention.

As if this is not bad enough, the bacteria can also break down protein via the process of putrefaction to produce what are known as *vasoactive amines.*[7] Vasoactive amines cause constriction and relaxation of blood vessels by acting on the smooth muscle that surrounds the vessels. In the intestinal tract, excessive vasoactive amine synthesis can lead to increased gut permeability (i.e., the leaky gut syndrome), abdominal pain, and altered gut motility. (Table 1.4 lists factors associated with small intestinal bacterial overgrowth.)

Symptoms of small intestinal bacterial overgrowth are similar to those generally attributed to chronic candidiasis as well as insufficient digestive secretions (lack of hydrochloric acid or pancreatic enzymes). Symptoms may also include more severe gastrointestinal symptoms such as nausea and diarrhea and arthritis. In fact, a study published in the *Annals of the Rheumatic Diseases* in 1993 demonstrated that many patients with rheumatoid arthritis exhibit small intestinal bacterial overgrowth and that the degree of overgrowth was associated with the severity of symptoms and disease activity.[8]

Diagnosis of small intestinal bacterial overgrowth involves careful evaluation of the CDSA (discussed above).

Table 1.4   Factors Associated with Small Intestinal Bacterial Overgrowth

Decreased digestive secretions

Achlorhydria (the complete absence of hydrochloric acid)

Hypochlorhydria (a defiency of hydrochloric acid)

Drugs that inhibit production of hydrochloric acid (such as Tagamet and Zantac)

Pancreatic insufficiency

Decreased bile output due to liver or gallbladder disease

Decreased motility (decrease in normal contractions of the gastrointestinal tract)

Scleroderma (progressive systemic sclerosis)

Systemic lupus erythematosus

Intestinal adhesions

Sugar-induced hypomotility

Radiation damage

Low secretory IgA

Weak ileocecal valve

There are also breath tests that measure the levels of hydrogen and methane after the administration of carbohydrates (lactulose and glucose). If there is small intestinal bacterial overgrowth, there will be higher than normal amounts of hydrogen and/or methane.

The treatment of small intestinal bacterial overgrowth is virtually identical to the treatment of chronic candidiasis. Specifically, the first step involves addressing and correcting the factors that predispose the individual to the bacterial or candida overgrowth. These factors are thoroughly discussed throughout this book.

The Leaky Gut Syndrome

Increased gastrointestinal permeability, a *leaky gut,* leads to absorption of large food particles, bacterial and yeast components, and various toxic chemicals. A leaky gut is one of the hallmark features of the yeast syndrome, but a leaky gut can be caused by overgrowth of *Candida albicans* as well as by other factors.

As a result of a leaky gut, a person may experience many symptoms often attributed to the yeast syndrome even though there is no overgrowth of *Candida albicans.* Other conditions linked to a leaky gut include: arthritis (both rheumatoid and osteoarthritis); autoimmune diseases such as Hashimoto's thyroiditis, scleroderma, systemic lupus erythematosus, and ankylosing spondylitis; cirrhosis of the liver (alcohol increases gut permeability); acne; psoriasis; and pancreatitis.[9–11] In addition, over 100 disorders, known as extra-intestinal lesions (EIL), constitute systemic complications of Crohn's disease and ulcerative colitis.[12–13] Increased gut permeability to due chronic inflammation is a hallmark feature of these conditions.

Diagnosing Leaky Gut Diagnosis of a leaky gut is fairly straightforward. It involves the administration of two sugars—mannitol and lactulose. Mannitol is a small sugar molecule that is quickly taken up by intestinal cells and transported into the system. Lactulose, on the other hand, is a larger molecule that should not be taken up by intestinal cells. However, if the junction between the intestinal cells is not tight (i.e., if it is leaky), lactulose will be absorbed. Therefore, mannitol serves as a marker for general absorption and lactulose serves as an indicator of increased intestinal permeability. Since neither sugar is metabolized, a six-hour urine measurement after administration of mannitol and lactulose is standard.

Normally, the percentage of mannitol that is recovered is between 5% to 25% and the percentage of lactulose that is recovered is 0.1% to 0.8%. If the levels of lactulose and mannitol are both increased, it indicates general increased intestinal permeability. If the levels of mannitol and lactulose are both decreased, it reflects malabsorption. And, if the level of lactulose is increased and the level of mannitol is decreased or the ratio of lactulose to mannitol is increased, it may indicate damage to absorptive surfaces similar to the damage associated with celiac disease.

In most circumstances, correcting the leaky gut requires addressing the same factors that can lead to the overgrowth of candida, bacterial overgrowth in the small intestine, chronic inflammation, and food allergies.

Final Comments

Because chronic candidiasis is truly a multifactorial condition, many factors must be taken into consideration regarding predisposing agents as well as treatment. This book is designed to provide a comprehensive overview of chronic candidiasis with the goal of identifying and effectively addressing the reasons for the candida overgrowth as well as the associated syndromes of small intestinal bacterial overgrowth and the leaky gut.

2

Antibiotics and
the Yeast Syndrome

Prolonged antibiotic use is believed to be the most important triggering factor in the development of chronic candidiasis in many cases. Antibiotics, by suppressing normal intestinal bacteria, which prevent yeast overgrowth and suppression of the immune system, strongly promote the overgrowth of candida.[1]

There is little argument that, when used appropriately, antibiotics save lives. Unfortunately, antibiotics are grossly overused. While the appropriate use of antibiotics makes good medical sense, what does not make sense is reliance on antibiotics to treat such conditions as acne, recurrent bladder infections, chronic ear infections, chronic sinusitis, chronic bronchitis, and non-bacterial sore throats. Relying on antibiotics to treat these conditions does not make sense for two reasons: (1) the antibiotics do not provide significant benefits and (2) these conditions can be effectively treated using natural measures.

When antibiotics are necessary, such as in the case of serious or potentially serious bacterial infections, they should be used in combination with an anti-fungal agent such as nystatin, Diflucan, or ketoconazole (all are discussed in Chapter 9) to combat the risk of developing a secondary yeast infection or overgrowth of candida in the gastro-intestinal or vaginal tract and *Lactobacillus acidophilus* (discussed in Chapter 8) to restore colonies of beneficial bacteria to the body.

Dependence Upon Antibiotics

Conventional medicine's dependence on antibiotics began when Louis Pasteur, a nineteenth-century physician and researcher, discovered the antibiotic effects of penicillin. Pasteur played a major role in the development of the germ theory. This theory holds that different diseases are caused by different infectious organisms. Much of Pasteur's life was dedicated to finding substances that would kill the infecting organisms. Pasteur and others since him who've pioneered effective treatments of infectious diseases have given us a great deal for which we should be thankful. However, there is more to the equation than the virility of the infecting organism.

Another nineteenth-century French scientist, Claude Bernard, also made major contributions to medical under-standing. But Bernard had a different view of health and disease. Bernard believed that the state of a person's internal environment, *milieu interieur,* was more important in determining disease than the invading organism. In other words, Bernard believed that the body's internal ter-rain or susceptibility to infection was more important than the germ. Physicians, he believed, should focus more of their attention on making this internal terrain a very in-hospitable place for disease.

Bernard's theory led to some rather interesting studies. In fact, a firm advocate of the germ theory would find some of these studies to be absolutely crazy. One of the most interesting studies was conducted by Elie Metchnikoff, a Russian scientist and the discoverer of white blood cells. He and his research associates consumed cultures containing millions of cholera bacteria. Yet none of them developed cholera. The reason: Their immune systems were not compromised. Metchnikoff believed, like Bernard, that the correct way to deal with infectious disease was to focus on enhancing the body's own defenses.

During the last part of their lives, Pasteur and Bernard engaged in scientific discussions on the virtues of the germ theory and Bernard's perspective on the internal terrain. On his deathbed, Pasteur said, "Bernard was right. The pathogen is nothing. The terrain is everything." Unfortunately, Pasteur's legacy is conventional medicine's obsession with the pathogen and the importance of the terrain has largely been forgotten.

Alternatives to Antibiotics

As stated previously, there are definite situations when antibiotics should be used. There is no question that antibiotics save lives. Yet antibiotics are widely used to treat conditions where they simply do not provide any real benefit or where natural measures can be used effectively and more safely. To illustrate some of the conditions where antibiotics provide little, if any, real benefits in most cases, let's look at their use in the treatment of bladder infections, respiratory tract infections, and acne.

Bladder Infections

Bladder infections are a very important factor to consider in treating the yeast syndrome because they are a common reason why women are placed on antibiotics. The typical symptoms of a bladder infection can include a burning pain on urination; increased urinary frequency; nighttime urination; a turbid, foul-smelling, or dark urine; and lower abdominal pain.

Most bladder infections are caused by bacteria, however the diagnosis of bladder infection by culturing the urine for bacteria is imprecise since clinical symptoms and the presence of significant amounts of bacteria in the urine do not always correlate well. Only 60% of women with the typical symptoms of urinary tract infection actually have significant levels of bacteria in their urine.

In general, the diagnosis is made according to signs and symptoms and urinary findings. Microscopic examination of the infected urine will show high levels of white blood cells and bacteria. Culturing the urine will determine the quantity and type of bacteria involved. *Escherichia coli* bacteria is responsible for about 90% of bladder infections.

Although most bladder infections are relatively benign, it is extremely important that they are properly diagnosed, treated, and monitored. Proper monitoring includes notifying a physician of any change in your condition. If an original urine culture was positive for bacteria, it is appropriate to follow-up with another culture 7 to 14 days after treatment was started.

Urine, as it is secreted by the kidneys, is sterile until it reaches the urethra. The urethra is the tube that transports the urine from the bladder to the urethral opening. Bacteria are introduced into the urethra by vaginal secretions.

The body has many natural defenses against bacterial growth in the urinary tract: urine flow tends to wash away bacteria, the surface of the bladder has anti-microbial properties, the pH of the urine inhibits the growth of many bacteria, and the body quickly secretes white blood cells to control the bacteria.

Using Antibiotics to Treat Bladder Infections

For most bladder infections, the best treatment appears to be the natural approach. There is a growing concern that antibiotic therapy actually promotes recurrent bladder infections by disturbing the bacterial flora of the vagina as well as promoting the growth of antibiotic-resistant strains of *E. coli*.[1,2] One of the most important ways in which the body prevents colonization of bacteria in the bladder is a protective shield of beneficial bacteria that line and protect the external portion of the urethra. When antibiotics are used, this normal protective shield is usually stripped away or is replaced by less effective organisms.

If you tend to suffer from recurrent bladder infections or if you have used antibiotics, it is important to reintroduce friendly bacteria into the vagina. The best way to do this is to use *Lactobacillus acidophilus* products, which are available at health food stores. Simply place one or two capsules or tablets in the vagina before going to bed at night. This practice should be continued for at least two weeks. (Refer to Chapter 8 for detailed discussion on the benefits of *Lactobacillus acidophilus.*)

The Natural Approach to Bladder Infections

The primary goal of the natural approach to treating bladder infections is enhancing normal host protective measures against urinary tract infections. Specifically this refers to enhancing the flow of urine by achieving and maintaining proper hydration, promoting a pH that will inhibit the growth of the organism, and preventing bacterial adherence to the endothelial cells of the bladder. In addition, there are several botanical medicines that can be employed.

Increasing Urine Flow   Increasing urine flow can be easily achieved simply by increasing the amount of liquids consumed. Ideally the liquids should be in the form of pure water, fresh juices diluted with an equal amount of water, and herbal teas. Drink at least 64 ounces of liquids from this group with at least half of this amount being water. Avoid liquids such as soft drinks, concentrated fruit drinks, coffee, and alcoholic beverages.

Of particular benefit in the treatment of urinary tract infections are cranberries. Cranberries and cranberry juice have been shown to be quite effective in several clinical studies.[3-5] In one study, 16 ounces of cranberry juice per day was shown to produce beneficial effects in 73% of the subjects (44 females and 16 males) with active urinary tract infections.[3] Furthermore, withdrawal of the cranberry juice in the people who benefited resulted in recurrence of bladder infection in 61%.

Although many people believe that the action of cranberry juice is due to its ability to acidify the urine in combination with the antibacterial effects of hippuric acid, a cranberry component, these are probably not the major mechanisms of action.[6,7] For example, in order to acidify the urine, at least 1 quart of cranberry juice would have to be consumed at one sitting. In addition, the concentration of hippuric acid in the urine as a result of drinking cranberry juice is not sufficient to inhibit bacteria.

However, drinking only 16 ounces of cranberry juice has been noted to have a positive effect in the treatment of bladder infection. This data indicates that another mechanism in the juice is more likely.

More recent studies have shown that components in cranberry juice reduce the ability of *E. coli* to stick to the mucosal lining of the bladder and urethra.[8,9] In order for bacteria to infect, they must first adhere to the mucosa. By interfering with adherence, cranberry juice greatly reduces the likelihood of infection and helps the body to fight off infection. This is the most likely explanation of cranberry juice's positive effects in treating bladder infections.

It must be pointed out that most cranberry juices on the market contain one-third cranberry juice mixed with water and sugar. Since sugar has such a detrimental effect on the immune system, use of sweetened cranberry juice cannot be recommended. Fresh cranberry (sweetened with apple or grape juice) or blueberry juice is preferred. Cranberry extracts are also available in pill form. The dosage of the cranberry extract should be based on the equivalent of 16 ounces of cranberry juice daily. There is no known toxicity as a result of cranberry ingestion.

Acidify or Alkalinize the Urine?   Although many physicians believe that acidifying the urine is the best approach in treating bladder infections, several arguments can be made for alkalinizing the urine instead. First of all, it is often very difficult to acidify the urine. Many popular methods of attempting to acidify the urine, such as ascorbic acid supplementation and the drinking of cranberry juice, have very little effect on pH at commonly prescribed doses.

The best argument for alkalinizing the urine is that it appears to be more effective than acidifying it, especially in women without evidence of bacteria in their urine. The best method for alkalinizing the urine appears to be the use of citrate salts, e.g., potassium citrate and sodium citrate. These salts are rapidly absorbed and metabolized without affecting gastric pH or producing a laxative effect. They are excreted partly as carbonate, thus raising the pH of the urine.

Potassium citrate and/or sodium citrate have long been employed in the treatment of lower urinary tract infections. They are often used as a "holding exercise" until the results of a urine culture are available. Clinical studies support this practice. For example, in one study, women with symptoms of a urinary tract infection were given a 4 g dose of sodium citrate every 8 hours for 48 hours.[10] Of the 64 women treated with the sodium citrate, 80% had relief of symptoms, 12% had deterioration of symptoms, and 91.8% rated the treatment as acceptable. Of the 64 women, 19 were shown to have a bacterial infection based upon the presence of bacteria in cultures. In the group of women with proven bacterial infection, symptoms of urethral pain and symptoms of painful urination improved more than urinary frequency and feelings of urgency. These results were very similar to another study that demonstrated significant symptomatic relief in 80% of the 159 women studied who did not have bacteria present in their urine.[11]

Another advantage to alkalinizing, rather than acidifying, the urine is that many of the herbs used to treat urinary tract infections, such as goldenseal and uva ursi, contain antibacterial components that work most effectively in an alkaline environment.

Rather than using potassium or sodium citrate alone, perhaps the best method of alkalinizing the urine is to take a multimineral formula where the minerals are bound (chelated) to citrate, malate, fumarate, or succinate. For example, in my clinical practice, I typically recommend that women with a bladder infection take two tablets of Krebs Cycle Chelates, made by Enzymatic Therapy, three times a day to help alkalinize their urine. This formula and similar formulas are available at health food stores.

Using Herbal Medicines   Many herbs have been used through the centuries in the treatment of urinary tract infections. The two with the greatest scientific support for their use are uva ursi (*Arctostaphylos uva ursi*), commonly called bearberry or upland cranberry, and goldenseal (*Hydrastis canadensis*).

Uva Ursi: Most research on uva ursi's urinary antiseptic properties has focused on arbutin, which typically composes 7% to 9% of the leaves. However, crude plant extracts are much more effective medicinally than isolated arbutin.[12] Uva ursi is reported to be especially active against *E. coli* and also has mild diuretic properties which help to evacuate the bladder.[13,14]

Care must be taken to avoid excessive dosages of uva ursi because little as 15 grams (½ ounce) of the dried leaves has been shown to produce toxicity in susceptible individuals. Toxic signs include ringing in the ears, nausea, vomiting, a sense of suffocation, shortness of breath, convulsions, delirium, and ultimately loss of consciousness.

Uva ursi is safe to use at the following dosage taken three times per day:

Dried leaves or as a tea: 1.5 to 4.0 g (approximately 1 to 2 tsp)

Tincture (1:5): 4 to 6 ml (1 to 1.5 tsp)

Fluid extract (1:1): 0.5 to 2.0 ml (¼ to ½ tsp)

Powdered solid extract (10% arbutin content): 250 to 500 mg

Goldenseal: Goldenseal is one of the most effective of the herbal anti-microbial agents. Its long history of use by herbalists and naturopathic physicians for the treatment of infections is well documented in the scientific literature.[15] Of particular importance in the treatment of bladder infections is its efficacy against most common bacteria, including *E. coli.*[15] Goldenseal's active ingredient, berberine, like uva ursi, works better in alkaline urine. Other berberine-containing plants such as Oregon grape root (*Berberis aquifolium*), barberry (*Berberis vulgaris*), and gold thread (*Coptis sinensis*) can be used interchangeably with goldenseal.

Goldenseal is safe to use at the following dosage taken three times per day:

Powdered dried root (in capsules) or as a tea: 1 to 2 g (roughly, 1 to 2 tsp)

Tincture (1:5): 4 to 6 ml (1 to 1.5 tsp)

Fluid extract (1:1): 0.5 to 2.0 ml (¼ to ½ tsp)

Powdered solid extract (8% alkaloid content): 250 to 500 mg

Treating Food Allergies   Food allergies are often a factor in producing the symptoms of a bladder infection.[16-18] If you suffer from symptoms of a bladder infection, yet there is no evidence of infection, it may be the result of food allergy. To treat food allergies, follow the dietary recommendations given in Chapter 4.

Antibiotics and Upper Respiratory Tract Infections

Most cases of sore throat (non-streptococcal pharyngitis), sinusitis, and/or bronchitis do not require antibiotics, yet many physicians prescribe antibiotics for these conditions in an attempt to help with symptoms and reduce the likelihood of secondary bacterial infection. However, there is little scientific support for this common practice. As an example, let's look at the use of antibiotics in the treatment of acute bronchitis.

Acute bronchitis, in general, refers to the acute onset of a productive cough in a patient with no history of asthma or chronic obstructive pulmonary disease and without evidence of pneumonia. Over the past 20 years, several randomized controlled trials have been designed to assess the benefit of antibiotics in treating acute bronchitis.[19,20] Despite substantial data showing no clinical benefit from antibiotics in treating acute bronchitis, these drugs are still prescribed by many doctors. Roughly 70% of doctors regularly prescribe an antibiotic to treat acute bronchitis even though it provides no benefit and significant risk. The risks include overgrowth of *Candida albicans,* disruption of normal gut microflora, and the possibility of developing antibiotic-resistant strains of bacteria.

Why then do physicians continue to prescribe antibiotics for acute bronchitis in light of the scientific facts? There are several misconceptions according to an editorial that appeared in the medical journal *The Lancet.*[20] Many doctors prescribe antibiotics when a patient's history is "I've had a cough for a week, and now my phlegm has turned green," even though the cough does not resolve any more quickly with the use of antibiotics than without. Likewise, many doctors use antibiotics because of a fever in acute bronchitis or in the hope of preventing potential progression to pneumonia, although the data do not support this strategy either.

Finally, doctors often prescribe antibiotics for acute bronchitis simply because many patients believe that only an antibiotic can cure it. This belief is perhaps best exemplified by a double-blind study, in which 60% of eligible patients refused to participate because they felt that antibiotics were absolutely necessary. Given these beliefs and expectations, it is little wonder that antibiotics continue to be prescribed for a condition in which they will not alter the course of the disease and thus are not warranted.

Treating Upper Respiratory Infections Naturally

Some natural alternatives to antibiotics for the treatment of upper respiratory infections are as follows:

Dietary and Lifestyle Guidelines

Avoid cigarette smoke and other respiratory irritants

Rest

Drink at least 48 ounces of water daily

Avoid sugar and dairy products

Supplement Protocol (Acute Treatment)

Thymus extract: 750 mg of the crude polypeptide fraction once or twice daily

Vitamin C: 500 to 1,000 mg every waking hour or to bowel tolerance (if excessive flatulence or diarrhea occurs, reduce dosage to a level that does not produce these symptoms)

Goldenseal root extract (8% to 10% berberine content): 400 mg three times daily on an empty stomach

Bromelain (see below): 400 mg three times daily on an empty stomach

Bromelain and Respiratory Tract Infections

Bromelain is a protein-digesting enzyme complex derived from pineapple, which has shown good results in the treatment of upper respiratory tract infections. For example, in the treatment of chronic bronchitis, bromelain was shown to have an anti-tussive (suppression of cough) effect and to reduce the thickness (viscosity) of sputum (mucolytic activity).

Examination of patients with a specialized apparatus for determining respiratory function (a spirometer) before and after treatment indicated increased lung capacity and function. These favorable effects were believed to be the results of enhanced resolution of respiratory congestion, due to bromelain's ability to fluidify and decrease bronchial secretions. It appears that bromelain's mucolytic activity is responsible for its particular effectiveness in treating respiratory tract diseases.[21]

Acute sinusitis has also responded to bromelain therapy. Good-to-excellent results were obtained in 87% of bromelain-treated patients, compared with 68% of the placebo group.[22]

Postural Drainage

In treating bronchitis, sinusitis, and pneumonia, one of the main goals is to help the lungs and air passages to get rid of the excessive mucus. I recommend that the following be performed twice daily: Apply a heating pad, hot water bottle, or a mustard poultice to the chest for up to 20 minutes. A mustard poultice is made by mixing one part dry mustard with three parts flour and adding enough water to make a paste. Spread the paste on thin cotton (an old pillowcase works well) or cheesecloth, folded, and then place on the chest. Check often because the mustard can cause blisters if left on too long.

After the hot pack, perform postural drainage by lying with the top half of your body off the bed using your forearms for support. The position should be assumed for a 5 to 15 minute period while trying to cough and expectorate into a basin or newspaper on the floor.

Acne

Acne is the most common of all skin problems. It occurs mostly on the face and, to a lesser extent, on the back, chest, and shoulders. Acne occurs in two forms: *acne vulgaris,* affecting the hair follicles and oil-secreting glands of the skin and manifesting as blackheads (comedones), whiteheads (pustules), and inflammation (papules) and *acne conglobata,* a more severe form, with deep cyst formation and subsequent scarring.

Tetracycline is the drug of choice of most dermatologists for the treatment of acne. It is generally thought to have fewer side effects and yield better results than other antibiotics. When tetracycline cannot be used due to intolerance or pregnancy, erythromycin is used. Tetracycline improves acne by preventing the overgrowth of bacteria in the skin pores. Tetracycline is most effective for the more superficial form of acne affecting the face.

The most common side effect of treatment with tetracycline is overgrowth of *Candida albicans* and other yeast in the gastrointestinal and genitourinary tracts. This can result in the appearance of symptoms attributed to chronic candidiasis as well as yeast infections of the mouth, intestinal tract, rectum, and/or vagina. Additional side effects are consistent with other antibiotics and include allergic reactions; nausea, diarrhea, and vomiting; loss of appetite; and colitis. In rare instances tetracycline can lead to anemia and low white blood cell and platelet levels.

Tetracycline is not used during pregnancy or lactation or in children under eight years of age because it interferes with tooth development. Use of tetracycline in these cases can result in permanent discoloration and/or malformation of teeth.

The Natural Approach to Acne

A healthful diet rich in natural whole foods such as vegetables, fruits, whole grains, and beans is the first recommendation for acne. All refined and/or concentrated sugars must be eliminated. Foods containing trans-fatty acids such as milk, milk products, margarine, shortening and other synthetically hydrogenated vegetable oils as well as fried foods must be avoided. Chocolate produces a double whammy in that it is high in both sugar and fats. Milk should be avoided not only because it contains trans-fatty acids, but also because it may contain trace levels of hormones. And, finally, foods high in iodized salt should be eliminated because some people are quite sensitive to the iodine, a known inducer of acne.

Here are seven additional recommendations:

1. Avoid medications that may cause acne:

    Anabolic steroids such as testosterone

    Corticosteroids

    Oral contraceptives

    Progesterone

    Drugs containing bromides or iodides

2. Avoid exposure to oils and greases

3. Avoid the use of greasy creams or cosmetics

4. Wash the pillowcase regularly in chemical-free (no added colors or fragrances) detergents

5. Remove excess sebum and oil from the face by washing thoroughly twice daily (more if necessary)

6. Take a high-potency multiple vitamin and mineral supplement according to the guidelines given in Chapter 5

7. Take 45 to 60 mg of zinc bound to either picolinate, citrate, or monomethionine

Zinc Versus Tetracycline

Several double-blind studies have demonstrated the effectiveness of zinc in the treatment of acne. In fact, these studies have shown zinc to yield similar results to tetracycline in superficial acne and superior results in deeper acne.[23–25] Although there are some studies of zinc in acne patients where improvements of this magnitude were not obtained, the inconsistency of the results can be explained by differences in dosages or the form of zinc used.

For example, studies using zinc citrate or zinc gluconate show improvements similar to tetracycline while those using plain zinc sulfate have shown less beneficial results, because zinc sulfate is poorly absorbed.[26,27] There have been no studies to date using other highly absorbable forms of zinc such as zinc picolinate, zinc acetate, or zinc monomethionine. These forms of zinc are more effectively absorbed than the forms of zinc used in the positive studies and, therefore, may produce even better effects. A safe and effective dose for zinc is 30 to 45 mg per day.

Although some people in these studies showed dramatic improvement immediately, the majority usually required 12 weeks of supplementation before good results were achieved.

Final Comments

The widespread use and abuse of antibiotics is alarming for many reasons besides the epidemic of chronic candidiasis. Excess use of antibiotics is encouraging the development of "superbugs," which are resistant to currently available antibiotics. According to many experts, as well as the World Health Organization, we are coming dangerously close to arriving at a "post-antibiotic era" where many infectious diseases will once again become almost impossible to treat.[28-30]

As stated earlier, antibiotics definitely have their place in modern medicine. However, there is a great need to avoid the use of antibiotics unless they are absolutely necessary. Inappropriate use greatly increases the risk of developing complications such as overgrowth of *Candida albicans* and other organisms as well as increasing the risk of developing a bacterial infection that is resistant to antibiotics—a very serious problem.

Antibiotic resistance is probably an inevitable process because bacteria transfer genetic material both within species and between species to help ensure survival of the organism. It has been well-demonstrated that antibiotic resistance is much more common where antibiotics are used more often.[29] A case in point is the hospital environment where infections caused by antibiotic-resistant strains of organisms such as *Staphylococcus aureus* and *Pseudomonas aeruginosa* often lead to fatal complications.

Since there is evidence that resistance to antibiotics is less of a problem when antibiotics are used sparingly, reduction in antibiotic prescriptions may be the only significant way to address the problem. According to the World Health Organization, as well as other scientific authorities, antibiotic use must be restricted and their inappropriate use halted if the growing trend toward bacterial resistance to antibiotics is to be stopped or reversed.[28-30] However, prescriptions for antibiotics are not the only source of concern: Antibiotics have been added to domestic animal feed since the 1950s.

It may be several more decades before it is truly known what effects the widespread use of antibiotics are having on many different health conditions. For example, antibiotic exposure is being linked to Crohn's disease.[31] Prior to the 1950s, Crohn's disease was found in selected groups with a strong genetic component. Since that time there has been a rapid climb in developed countries, particularly in the United States, and in countries that previously had virtually no reported cases. In fact, since 1950 Crohn's disease has spread like an epidemic.

Are antibiotics to blame? Penicillin and tetracycline have been available in oral form since 1953. The annual increase in prescriptions of antibiotics and the fact that there is a parallel increase in the annual incidence of

Crohn's disease is harrowing. Comparative statistics have shown that wherever antibiotics were used early and in large quantities, the incidence of Crohn's disease is now quite high.

Over the years researchers have sought to identify Crohn's disease as an infectious process. Frighteningly, the infectious agent may be a component of the normal intestinal flora, which suddenly produces immuno-stimulatory toxins or becomes invasive as a direct result of sub-lethal doses of antibiotics. Administration of sub-lethal amounts of antibiotics has been shown to induce a capacity for toxin production in intestinal organisms. When microbes are not given a full lethal dose, their usual response is to adapt and become even stronger and more numerous.

The bottom line is that antibiotic use should not be viewed casually. Try to avoid using antibiotics unless absolutely necessary.

3

Enhancing
Digestive Secretions

Digestive secretions—such as gastric hydrochloric acid, pancreatic enzymes, and bile—inhibit the overgrowth of candida and prevent its penetration into the absorptive surfaces of the small intestine. Decreased secretion of any of these important digestive components can lead to overgrowth of *Candida albicans* in the gastrointestinal tract. Therefore, restoration of normal digestive secretions through the use of supplemental hydrochloric acid, pancreatic enzymes, and substances that promote bile flow is critical in the treatment of chronic candidiasis. The CSDA (see Chapter 1) can provide valuable information in identifying the most important factors.

Hypochlorhydria and Candidiasis

Patients on anti-ulcer drugs such as Tagamet (cimetidine) and Zantac (ranitidine), which inhibit the production of hydrochloric acid, actually develop candida overgrowth in the stomach.[1] This occurrence highlights the importance of hydrochloric acid in the prevention of candida overgrowth. Although much is said about hyperacidity conditions, probably a more common cause of indigestion is a *lack* of gastric acid secretion. *Hypochlorhydria* refers to deficient gastric acid secretion while *achlorhydria* refers to a complete absence of gastric acid secretion.

Impaired gastric acid secretion displays many symptoms and signs which are listed in Table 3.1. Also, a number of specific diseases have been found to be associated with insufficient gastric acid output, these are listed in Table 3.2.[2-13]

The best method of diagnosing of a lack of gastric acid is a special procedure known as the *Heidelberg gastric analysis*.[14] This technique utilizes an electronic capsule attached to a string. The capsule is swallowed and then kept in the stomach with the aid of the string. The capsule measures the pH of the stomach and sends a radio message to a receiver, which then records the pH level. Dr. Jonathan Wright believes that the response to a bicarbonate challenge during Heidelberg gastric analysis is the true test of the functional ability of the stomach to secrete acid.[15] After the test, the capsule is removed from the stomach by the string attached to it.

Since not everyone can have detailed gastric acid analysis to determine their need for gastric acid supplementation, a more practical method of determination is often used. If an individual is experiencing any signs and symptoms of gastric acid insufficiency as listed in Table 3.1 or has any of the diseases listed in Table 3.2 the method as outlined below can be employed.

Protocol for Hydrochloric Acid Supplements

1. Begin by taking one tablet or capsule containing 10 grains (600 mg) of hydrochloric acid at your next

Table 3.1   Common Signs and Symptoms of
Low Gastric Acidity

Bloating, belching, burning, and flatulence immediately after meals	Dilated blood vessels in the cheeks and nose
A sense of "fullness" after eating	Acne
Indigestion, diarrhea, or constipation	Iron deficiency
Multiple food allergies	Chronic intestinal parasites or abnormal flora
Nausea after taking supplements	Undigested food in stool
Itching around the rectum	Chronic candida infections
Weak, peeling, and cracked fingernails	Upper digestive tract gassiness

Table 3.2   Diseases Associated with Low Gastric Acidity

Addison's disease	Lupus erythematosus
Asthma	Myasthenia gravis
Celiac disease	Osteoporosis
Dermatitis herpetiformis	Pernicious anemia
Diabetes mellitus	Psoriasis
Eczema	Rheumatoid arthritis
Gallbladder disease	Rosacea
Graves disease	Sjogren's syndrome
Chronic auto-immune disorders	Thyrotoxicosis
Hepatitis	Hyper- and hypothyroidism
Chronic hives	Vitiligo

large meal. If this does not aggravate your symptoms, at every meal after that of the same size take one more tablet or capsule. (One at the next meal, two at the meal after that, then three at the next meal.)

2. Continue to increase the dose until you reach seven tablets or when you feel a warmth in your stomach, whichever occurs first. A feeling of warmth in the stomach means that you have taken too many tablets for that meal, and you need to take one less tablet for that meal size. It is a good idea to try the larger dose again at another meal to make sure that it was the HCl that caused the warmth and not something else.

3. After you have found the largest dose that you can take at your large meals without feeling any warmth, maintain that dose at all of meals of similar size. You will need to take less at smaller meals.

4. When taking a number of tablets or capsules it is best to take them throughout the meal.

5. As your stomach begins to regain the ability to produce the amount of HCl needed to properly digest your food, you will notice the warm feeling again and will have to cut down the dosage. HCl may be used indefinitely.

The Pancreas

The pancreas produces enzymes that are required for the digestion and absorption of food. Each day the pancreas secretes about 1.5 quarts of pancreatic juice in the small intestine. Enzymes secreted include lipases, proteases, and amylases. Lipases, along with bile, function in the digestion of fats. Amylases break down starch molecules into smaller sugars. The proteases secreted by the pancreas (trypsin, chymotrypsin, and carboxypeptidase) function in digestion by breaking down protein molecules into single amino acids. Incomplete digestion of proteins creates a number of problems for the body including the development of allergies and formation of toxic substances produced during putrefaction. Putrefaction refers to the breakdown of protein material by bacteria.

Pancreatin in the Treatment of the Yeast Syndrome

Pancreatic enzymes (proteases) can be quite useful in the treatment of chronic candidiasis. As well as being necessary for protein digestion, the proteases serve several other important functions. The proteases are largely responsible for keeping the small intestine free from parasites (including bacteria, yeast, protozoa, and intestinal worms).[16,17] A lack of proteases or other digestive secretions greatly increases an individual's risk of contracting an intestinal infection, including chronic candida infections of the gastrointestinal tract.

Assessing Pancreatic Function

Nutrition-oriented physicians use both physical symptoms and laboratory tests to assess pancreatic function. Common symptoms of pancreatic insufficiency include abdominal bloating and discomfort, gas, indigestion, and the passing of undigested food in the stool. For laboratory diagnosis, most nutrition-oriented physicians use the CSDA (discussed in Chapter 1).

Pancreatic insufficiency is characterized by impaired digestion, malabsorption of nutrients, nutrient deficiencies, and abdominal discomfort. The most severe level of pancreatic insufficiency is seen in cystic fibrosis, an inherited disorder. Although cystic fibrosis is quite rare, mild pancreatic insufficiency is thought to be a relatively common condition, especially in the elderly.

Pancreatic enzyme products are the most effective treatment for pancreatic insufficiency and are also quite popular digestive aids. Most commercial preparations are prepared from fresh hog pancreas (pancreatin).

Dosage for Pancreatic Enzymes   Even in the absence of pancreatic insufficiency as determined by the CSDA, I often recommend the use of pancreatic enzymes in patients with the yeast syndrome. The reason is that these enzymes appear to help rid the body of yeast cells as well as deal more effectively with any food allergies.

In order for a food molecule to produce an allergic response it must be a fairly large molecule. In studies performed in the 1930s and 1940s, pancreatic enzymes were shown to be quite effective in preventing food allergies.[18] It appears that many practitioners are not aware of, or have forgotten about, these early studies. Typically individuals who do not secrete enough proteases suffer from multiple food allergies.

The dosage of pancreatic enzymes is based on the level of enzyme activity of the particular product. The United States Pharmacopoeia (USP) has set a strict definition for level of activity. A 1X pancreatic enzyme (pancreatin) product has in each milligram not less than 25 USP units of amylase activity, not less than 2.0 USP units of lipase activity, and not less than 25 USP units of protease activity.

Pancreatin of higher potency is given a whole-number multiple indicating its strength. For example, a full-strength undiluted pancreatic extract that is 10 times stronger than the USP standard would be referred to as 10X USP. Full-strength products are preferred to lower potency pancreatin products because lower potency products are often diluted with salt, lactose, or galactose to achieve desired strength (e.g., 4X or 1X).

The dosage recommendation for a 10X USP pancreatic enzyme product in the treatment of chronic candidiasis would be 350 to 1,000 mg three times a day immediately before meals.

Enzyme products are often enteric-coated, that is they are often coated to prevent digestion in the stomach, so that the enzymes will be liberated in the small intestine. However, numerous studies have shown that non-enteric-coated enzyme preparations actually outperform enteric-coated products if they are given prior to a meal (for digestive purposes) or on an empty stomach (for anti-inflammatory effects).

Final Comments

My clinical experience is that impaired digestive secretions, usually a lack of both hydrochloric acid and pancreatic enzymes, are common in patients with chronic candidiasis. Again, the CSDA can be invaluable in providing this information. However, it is not entirely necessary.

If you appear to be suffering from hypochlorhydria, try the challenge protocol described above. If after determining your optimum dosage, you have not found any real benefit, try taking pancreatin as described above before meals in addition to the hydrochloric acid. If you still do not experience any significant benefit, I definitely recommend consulting a physician.

4

Dietary Factors

A number of dietary factors appear to promote the overgrowth of candida. The most important contributing factors are a high intake of sugar, milk and other dairy products, foods containing a high content of yeast or mold, and food allergies. Discussion of these factors will be followed by concise dietary recommendations for treating the yeast syndrome.

Sugar and the Yeast Syndrome

Sugar is the chief nutrient of *Candida albicans*. It is well-accepted that restriction of sugar intake is an absolute necessity in the treatment of chronic candidiasis. Most patients do well by simply avoiding refined sugar and large amounts of honey, maple syrup, and fruit juice.[1-4]

A Closer Look at Sugars

Sugars (carbohydrates) are divided into two primary categories: simple sugars and complex carbohydrates. Simple sugars are either monosaccharides composed of one sugar molecule or disaccharides composed of two sugar molecules. The principle monosaccharides that occur in foods are glucose and fructose. The major disaccharides are sucrose (white sugar), which is composed of one molecule of glucose and one molecule of fructose; maltose (glucose and glucose); and lactose (glucose and galactose).

Simple sugars are quickly absorbed by the body for a ready source of energy. It is thought by many that the assortment of natural simple sugars in fruits and vegetables have an advantage over sucrose (white sugar) and other refined sugars in that they are balanced by a wide range of nutrients that aid in the utilization of the sugars. Problems with carbohydrates really begin when they are refined and stripped of these nutrients. Virtually all of the vitamin content has been removed from white sugar, white breads, and pastries, and many breakfast cereals. Nonetheless, in patients with severe chronic candidiasis it is important to restrict all simple sugars even those from fruits, fruit juices, and high-sugar vegetable juices such as carrot.

Read food labels carefully for clues on sugar content. If the words *sucrose, glucose, maltose, lactose, fructose, corn syrup,* or *white grape juice concentrate* appear on the label, extra sugar has been added. Currently, more than half of the carbohydrates being consumed by people in the United States are in the form of sugars added to foods as sweetening agents.

Complex carbohydrates, or starches, are composed of many simple sugars joined together by chemical bonds. The body breaks down complex carbohydrates into simple sugars gradually, which leads to better blood sugar control. Complex carbohydrates are usually well-tolerated by patients with chronic candidiasis. In fact, the ingestion of fiber-rich complex-carbohydrate foods such as vegetables, legumes, and grains is very important in the treatment of candidiasis because it leads to a more favorable gastrointestinal bacterial flora. I encourage regular consumption of these foods.

Milk and Dairy Products

There are several reasons to restrict or eliminate the intake of milk in patients with chronic candidiasis: (1) the high lactose content promotes the overgrowth of candida; (2) milk is one of the most frequent food allergens; and (3) milk may contain trace levels of antibiotics, which can further disrupt the gastrointestinal bacterial flora and promote candida overgrowth.[1-4]

Mold- and Yeast-Containing Foods

It is generally recommended by many experts that individuals with chronic candidiasis avoid foods with a high content of yeast or mold, including alcoholic beverages, cheeses, dried fruits, and peanuts. Even though many patients with chronic candidiasis may be able to tolerate these foods, I think it is still a good idea to eliminate them from the diet. At the very least they should be avoided until the candidiasis is under control.[1-4]

Food Allergies

Food allergies are another common finding in patients with the yeast syndrome.[3] A food allergy occurs when there is an adverse reaction to the ingestion of a food. The reaction may or may not be mediated by the immune system. The reaction may be caused by a food protein, starch, or other food component, or by a contaminant found in the food (colorings, preservatives, etc.). A classic food allergy occurs when an ingested food molecule acts as an *antigen,* which is defined as a substance that can be bound by antibodies known as IgE. IgE then binds to specialized white blood cells known as *mast cells* and *basophils.* This binding causes the release of substances such as histamine, which cause swelling and inflammation.

Other words often used to refer to a food allergy include *food hypersensitivity, food anaphylaxis, food idiosyncrasy, food intolerance, pharmacological (drug-like) reaction to food, metabolic reaction to food,* and *food sensitivity.* From a clinical perspective, naturopaths, clinical ecologists, and preventive- and nutrition-oriented physicians recognize two basic types of food allergies—cyclic and fixed.

Cyclic allergies account for 80% to 90% of food allergies. The sensitivity is slowly developed by repetitive eating of a food. If the allergic food is avoided for a period of time (typically over four months), it may be reintroduced and tolerated unless it is again eaten too frequently.

Fixed allergies occur whenever a food is eaten, no matter what the time span is between ingestions. Long-term avoidance may reestablish tolerance, but it is no guarantee.

Signs and Symptoms of Food Allergies

Food allergies have been implicated as a causative factor in a wide range of conditions; no part of the human body is immune from being a target. The actual symptoms produced during an allergic response depend on the location of the immune-system activation, the mediators of inflammation involved, and the sensitivity of the tissues to specific mediators. As shown in Table 4.1, food allergies have been linked to many common symptoms and health conditions.

The number of people suffering from food allergies has increased dramatically during the last 15 years. Some physicians claim that food allergies are the leading cause of most undiagnosed symptoms and that at least 60% of the U.S. population suffers from symptoms associated with food reactions.[5] Theories of why the incidence has increased include increased stresses on the immune system (such as greater chemical pollution in the air, water, and food), earlier weaning and earlier introduction of solid foods to infants, genetic manipulation of plants resulting in food components with greater allergenic tendencies, and increased ingestion of fewer foods. Probably all of these and more have contributed to the increased frequency and severity of symptoms.

Table 4.1   Symptoms and Diseases Commonly Associated with Food Allergies

System	Symptoms and Diseases
Gastrointestinal	canker sores, celiac disease, chronic diarrhea, stomach ulcer, gas, gastritis, irritable colon, malabsorption, ulcerative colitis
Genitourinary	bed-wetting, chronic bladder infections, kidney disease
Immune	chronic infections, frequent ear infections
Mental/Emotional	anxiety, depression, hyperactivity, inability to concentrate, insomnia, irritability, mental confusion, personality change, seizures
Musculoskeletal	bursitis, joint pain, low back pain
Respiratory	asthma, chronic bronchitis, wheezing
Skin	acne, eczema, hives, itching, skin rash
Miscellaneous	arrythmia, edema, fainting, fatigue, headache, hypoglycemia, itchy nose or throat, migraines, sinusitis

Food allergies, as well as respiratory tract allergies, are also characterized by the following signs:

Dark circles under the eyes (allergic shiners)

Puffiness under the eyes

Horizontal creases in the lower lid

Chronic noncyclic fluid retention

Chronic swollen glands

It is often not clearly apparent that a symptom is due to a food allergy perhaps because the body adapts to chronic exposure to allergenic foods. According to Theron Randolph, M.D., the symptom process may involve the following three stages:

Stage 1—Hypersensitivity (pre-adapted): Obvious allergic response following exposure to allergenic food.

Stage 2—Adaptive: Less recognizable response after eating the allergenic food and an increase in chronic symptoms. This can be considered an addictive phase, since ingestion of the allergenic food(s) may actually temporarily relieve symptoms. This stage typically involves food cravings and withdrawal responses. This is also known as *masked allergies.*

Stage 3—Maladaptive: The body is in a constant state of biochemical dysfunction. The allergic person is totally unaware of sensitivities as a cause of their ill health.[6]

What Causes Food Allergies?

It is well-documented that food allergy is often inherited. When both parents have allergies, there is a 67% chance that the children will also have allergies. Where only one parent is allergic, the chance of a child being prone to allergies drops to 33%.[7] The actual expression of an allergy can be triggered by a variety of stressors that disrupt the immune system, such as physical and emotional trauma, excessive use of drugs, immunization reactions, excessive frequency of consumption of a specific food, and environmental toxins.

Most food allergies are mediated by the immune system as a result of interactions between ingested food, the digestive tract, white blood cells, and food-specific antibodies (immunoglobulins). Food molecules capable of being bound by antibodies are known as *antigens.* Food represents the largest antigenic challenge confronting the human immune system. When the immune system is activated by food antigens, white blood cells and antibodies cooperate in an immune response, which, under certain circumstances, can have negative effects.

There are five major families of antibodies: IgE, IgD, IgG, IgM, and IgA. IgE is involved primarily in the classic immediate allergic reaction, while the others seem to be involved in delayed reactions, such as those seen in the cyclic type of food allergy. Although the function of the immune system is protection of the host from infections and cancer, abnormal immune responses can lead to tissue injury and disease (food allergy reactions being one expression). There are four distinct types of immune-mediated reactions: immediate hypersensitivity, cytotoxic reactions, immune-complex mediated reactions, and T-cell dependent reactions.

Immediate Hypersensitivity

With immediate hypersensitivity, the reactions occur in less than 2 hours after exposure to the allergen. Antigens bind to pre-formed IgE antibodies attached to the surface of the mast cell or the basophil and cause release of mediators:

histamine, leukotrienes, and so on. A variety of allergic symptoms may result, depending on the location of the mast cell: In the nasal passages it causes sinus congestion; in the bronchioles, constriction (asthma); in the skin, hives and eczema; in the synovial cells that line the joints, arthritis; in the intestinal mucosa, inflammation with resulting malabsorption; and in the brain, headaches, loss of memory, and "spaciness." It has been estimated that immediate hypersensitivity reactions account for only 10% to 15% of food allergy reactions.[8]

Cytotoxic Reactions

Cytotoxic reactions involve the binding of either IgG or IgM antibodies to cell-bound antigens. Antigen–antibody binding activates factors that result in the destruction of the cell to which the antigen is bound. Examples of tissue injury include immune hemolytic anemia. It has been estimated that at least 75% of all food allergy reactions are accompanied by cell destruction.[8]

Immune-Complex Mediated Reactions

Immune complexes are formed when antigens bind to antibodies. They are usually cleared from the circulation by the phagocytic system. However, if these complexes are deposited in tissues they can produce tissue injury. Two important factors that promote tissue injury are (1) increased quantities of circulating complexes and (2) the presence of histamine and other amines, which increase vascular permeability and favor the deposition of immune complexes in tissues.

These responses are of the delayed type, often occurring more than 2 hours after exposure. This type of allergy has been shown to involve IgG and IgG immune complexes. It is estimated that 80% of food allergy reactions involve IgG.[8]

T-Cell Dependent Reactions

This delayed type of reaction is mediated primarily by T-lymphocytes. It results when an allergen contacts the skin, respiratory tract, gastrointestinal tract, or some other body surface. Within 36 to 72 hours of contact, it can cause inflammation by stimulating sensitized T-cells. T-cell dependent reactions do not involve any antibodies. An example of this type of reaction is poison ivy (contact dermatitis).

Immune-System Disorders and Food Allergies

Several immune-system disorders can play a major role in food allergies. For example, some studies have shown that individuals with a tendency to develop asthma and eczema have abnormalities in the number and ratios of T-cells. Specifically, these individuals have nearly 50% more helper T-cells than nonallergic persons.[8] These cells help other white blood cells make antibodies.

An emerging theory suggests that individuals prone to asthma and eczema have a lower allergic set point. With more helper T-cells in circulation, the level of attack required to trigger an allergic response is lowered. Other T-cell abnormalities have been noted in patients with migraines and in asthmatic children; both groups commonly suffer from food allergies.[5]

Food-sensitive people usually have unusually low levels of secretory IgA.[9] IgA plays an important role on the lining of the mucosal membrane surfaces of the intestinal tract, where it helps protect against the entrance of foreign substances into the body. In other words, IgA acts as a barricade against the entry of food antigens. When there is a lack of IgA lining the intestines, the absorption of food allergens as well as microbial antigens increases dramatically. It has been suggested that even a short-term IgA deficiency predisposes one to the development of allergy, especially during the first months of life.

There is also evidence that stress can impair immune function and lead to decreased secretory IgA.[10] These findings might explain the relationship that many observers report between food allergy and stress. During stress, food allergies tend to be more apparent and, as a result, symptoms of chronic candidiasis tend to increase in severity.

Other Factors Triggering Food Allergies

Repetitious exposure to a food, improper digestion, and poor integrity of the intestinal barrier are additional factors that can lead to the development of food allergies. When properly chewed and digested, 98% of ingested proteins are absorbed as amino acids and small peptides. However, it has been well-documented that partially digested dietary protein can cross the intestinal barrier and be absorbed into the bloodstream. It then causes a food-allergic response, which can occur directly at the intestinal barrier, at distant sites, or throughout the body.

Gastric acidity and pancreatic enzymes limit the passage of organisms into the intestinal tract and are important in the digestion of protein. Low hydrochloric-acid and pancreatic-enzyme levels are associated with an increased incidence of intestinal infections and increased circulating antibodies to foods. It is often necessary to support the individual with food allergies with supplemental levels of hydrochloric acid and/or pancreatic enzymes because incompletely digested proteins can impair the immune system, leading to long-term allergies.

In addition to lack of essential digestive elements, other causes of an increased intestinal absorption of large protein molecules include immaturity of the gastrointestinal system, abnormal bacteria in the gut, vitamin A deficiency, inflammation of the intestinal tract, intestinal ulceration, and diarrhea. Proper functioning of the liver is also very important due to its role in removing foreign proteins.

Nonimmunological Mechanisms

Many adverse reactions to foods are not triggered by the immune system. Instead, the reaction is caused by inflammatory mediators (prostaglandins, leukotrienes, SRS-A, serotonin, platelet-activating factor, histamine, kinins, etc.). Foods may also produce a pseudo-allergic reaction (see Table 4.2) due to histamine content or histamine-releasing effects and reactions to compounds in foods known as

Table 4.2   Mechanisms Responsible for
Pseudo-Allergic Reactions

Increased production of inflammatory mediators.

Activation of platelets resulting in serotonin release.

Enhanced reactivity of mast cells and/or basophils to various triggering stimuli.

Excessive intake of histamine-containing foods—sausage, sauerkraut, tuna, wine, preserves, spinach, tomato.

Excessive intake of histamine-releasing foods—mollusks, crustaceans, strawberry, tomato, chocolate, protease-containing fruits (bananas, papaya), lecithin-containing nuts, peptones, alcohol.

Intolerance to foods containing vasoactive amines—tyramine (cabbage, cheese, citrus, seafood, potato), serotonin (banana), phenylethyl-amine (chocolate).

biogenic amines, including such compounds as tyramine, serotonin, and polyamines.

Diagnosis of Food Allergy

Two basic categories of tests are commonly used to diagnose food allergy: (1) food challenge and (2) laboratory methods. Each has its advantages. Food-challenge methods require no additional expense, but do require a great deal of motivation. Laboratory procedures, such as blood tests, can provide immediate identification of suspected allergens, but are more expensive.

Food Challenge

Many physicians believe that oral food challenge is the best way of diagnosing food sensitivities. There are two broad categories of food challenge testing: (1) elimination (also known as oligoantigenic) diet, followed by food reintroduction, and (2) pure water fast, followed by food challenge. A note of caution, food-challenge testing should *not* be used in people with symptoms that are potentially life-threatening (such as airway constriction or severe allergic reactions).

In the elimination-diet method, the person is placed on a limited diet; commonly eaten foods are eliminated and replaced with either hypoallergenic foods and foods rarely eaten or special hypoallergenic formulas.[11,12] The fewer the allergenic foods, the greater the ease of establishing a diagnosis with an elimination diet. The standard elimination diet consists of lamb, chicken, potato, rice, banana, apple, and a cabbage-family vegetable (cabbage, brussels sprouts, broccoli, etc.). There are variations of the elimination diet that are suitable, however, it is extremely important that no allergenic foods be consumed.

The individual stays on this limited diet for at least one week and up to one month. If the symptoms are related to food sensitivity, they will typically disappear by the fifth or sixth day of the diet. If the symptoms do not disappear, it is possible that a reaction to a food in the elimination diet is responsible, in which case an even more restricted diet must be utilized.

After one week, individual foods are reintroduced. Methods range from reintroducing only a single food every two days, to one every one or two meals. Usually after the one week "cleansing" period, the patient will develop an increased sensitivity to offending foods.

Reintroduction of sensitive foods will typically produce a more severe or recognizable symptom than before. A careful, detailed record must be maintained that describes when foods were reintroduced and what symptoms appeared upon reintroduction.[13] It can be very useful to track the wrist pulse during reintroduction, as pulse changes may occur when an allergenic food is consumed.[14]

For many people, elimination diets offer the most viable means of detection. Because one can sometimes dramatically experience the effects of food reactions, motivation to eliminate the food can be high. The downside of this procedure is that it is time-consuming and requires discipline and motivation.

A refinement, which often yields better results than the simple elimination diet, is the five-day water fast with subsequent food challenge. Proponents of this approach believe that it is necessary for the patient to fast for at least five days in order to clear the body of allergic responses.[15] During the fast, "withdrawal" symptoms such as intense cravings for allergenic foods and/or worsening of symptoms will likely be experienced. As in the elimination diet, symptoms caused by food allergy will diminish or be eliminated after the fourth day.

After the five-day fast, individual foods are reintroduced one at a time, with the monitoring of symptoms and pulse. Due to the hyperreactive state, symptoms tend to be more acute and pronounced than before the fast. This method can produce dramatic results, greatly motivating avoidance of the offending foods.

This method is advisable only for people who are physically and mentally capable of a five-day water fast. Close monitoring by a physician with experience in fasting is highly recommended. At times, careful interpretation of results is needed, due to the occurrence of delayed reactions.

Laboratory Methods

Laboratory methods for detecting food allergies consist of either skin or blood tests.

Skin Tests   It must be pointed out that the skin-prick test or skin-scratch test commonly employed by many allergists only tests for IgE-mediated allergies. Because only about 10% to 15% of all food allergies are mediated by IgE, this test is of little value in diagnosing most food allergies. Nonetheless, skin tests are often performed.

Food extracts are placed on the patient's skin with a scratch or prick. If the patient is allergic to the food, a welt will form immediately as the allergen reacts with IgE-sensitized cells in the patient's skin.

Blood Tests   Despite a tremendous amount of scientific support, the diagnosis of food allergy by blood testing is still somewhat controversial in conventional medical settings. These tests are convenient, but can range in cost from a modest $85 to an extravagant $1,200. A variety of blood tests are available to physicians with the RAST (radio-allergo-sorbent test) and the ELISA (enzyme-linked immunosorbent assay) test appearing to be the best laboratory methods currently available. In my clinical practice, I tend to favor the ELISA tests, which determine both IgE- and IgG-mediated food allergies. Laboratories that I would recommend for this analysis are National BioTech Laboratory (1-800-846-6285) and Meridian Valley Clinical Laboratory (1-206-859-8700). These laboratories offer IgE and IgG food-allergy panel tests for over 100 different foods; the test results come with detailed dietary instructions and are reasonably priced at about $85 to $170.

Dealing with Food Allergies

While there is no known simple "cure" for food allergies, a number of measures will help to avoid and lessen symptoms and can correct the underlying causes. First, all allergenic foods should be identified using one of the methods discussed above. After identifying allergenic foods, the best approach is clearly avoidance of all major allergens, and rotation of all other foods for at least the first few months. As one improves, the dietary restrictions can be relaxed, although some individuals may always require a rotation diet. For strongly allergenic foods, all members of the food family should be avoided.

Avoiding Allergenic Foods

The simplest and most effective method of treating food allergies is through avoidance of allergenic foods. Elimination of the offending antigens from the diet will begin to alleviate associated symptoms after the body has cleared itself of the antigen–antibody complexes and after the intestinal tract has transited out any remaining food (usually three to five days). Avoidance means not only avoiding the food in its most identifiable state (e.g., eggs in an omelet), but also in its hidden state (e.g., eggs in bread).

For severe reactions, closely related foods with similar antigenic components may also need to be eliminated (e.g., rice and millet in patients with severe wheat allergy).

However, avoiding allergenic foods may not be practical, for several reasons:

1. Common allergenic foods such as wheat, corn, and soy are found as components of many processed foods.

2. When eating away from home, it is often difficult to determine what ingredients are used in purchased foods and prepared meals.

3. There has been a dramatic increase in the number of foods that single individuals are allergic to. This condition represents a syndrome that is possibly indicative of broad immune-system dysfunction. It may be difficult (psychologically, socially, and nutritionally) to eliminate a large number of common foods from a person's diet.

A possible solution is the Rotary Diversified Diet.

Rotary Diversified Diet

Many experts believe that the key to the dietary control of food allergies is the *Rotary Diversified Diet*. The diet was first developed by Dr. Herbert J. Rinkel in 1934.[16] The diet is made up of a highly varied selection of foods, which are eaten in a definite rotation, or order, to prevent the formation of new allergies and to control preexisting ones.

Tolerated foods are eaten at regularly spaced intervals of four to seven days. For example, if a person has wheat on Monday, she will have to wait until Friday to have anything with wheat in it again. This approach is based on the principle that infrequent consumption of tolerated foods is not likely to induce new allergies or increase any mild allergies, even in highly sensitized and immune-compromised individuals. As tolerance for eliminated foods returns, they may be added back into the rotation schedule without reactivation of the allergy (this of course applies only to cyclic food allergies—fixed allergenic foods may never be eaten again).

It is not simply a matter of rotating tolerated foods; food families must also be rotated. Foods, whether animal or vegetable, come in families. The reason it is important to rotate food families is that foods in one family can cross-react with allergenic foods. Steady consumption of foods that are members of the same family can lead to allergies. Food families need not be as strictly rotated as individual foods. It is usually recommended to avoid eating members of the same food family two days in a row. Table 4.3 lists family classifications for edible plants and animals while a simplified four-day rotation diet plan is provided in Table 4.4.

Table 4.3 Edible Plant and Animal Kingdom Taxonomic List

		Vegetables		
Legumes	**Mustard**	**Parsley**	**Potato**	**Grass**
Beans	Broccoli	Anise	Chili	Barley
Cocoa bean	Brussels sprout	Caraway	Eggplant	Corn
Lentil	Cabbage	Carrot	Peppers	Oat
Licorice	Cauliflower	Celery	Potatoes	Rice
Peanut	Mustard	Coriander	Tomato	Rye
Peas	Radish	Cumin	Tobacco	Wheat
Soybean	Turnip	Parsley		
Tamarind	Watercress			
Lily	**Laurel**	**Sunflower**	**Beet**	**Buckwheat**
Asparagus	Avocado	Artichoke	Beet	Buckwheat
Chives	Camphor	Lettuce	Chard	Rhubarb
Garlic	Cinnamon	Sunflower	Spinach	
Leek				
Onions				

Continued

Table 4.3   Edible Plant and Animal Kingdom Taxonomic List
(continued)

Fruits

Gourds	Plums	Citrus	Cashew	Nuts
Cantaloupe	Almond	Grapefruit	Cashew	Brazil nut
Cucumber	Apricot	Lemon	Mango	Pecan
Honeydew	Cherry	Lime	Pistachio	Walnut
Melons	Peach	Mandarin		
Pumpkin	Plum	Orange		
Squash	Persimmon	Tangerine		
Zucchini				

Beech	Banana	Palm	Grape	Pineapple
Beechnut	Arrowroot	Coconut	Grape	Pineapple
Chestnut	Banana	Date	Raisin	
Chinquapin nut	Plantain	Date sugar		

Rose	Birch	Apple	Blueberry	Pawpaw
Blackberry	Filberts	Apple	Blueberry	Papaya
Loganberry	Hazelnuts	Pear	Cranberry	Pawpaw
Raspberry		Quince	Huckleberry	
Rosehips				
Strawberry				

Animals

Mammals (Meat/Milk)	Birds (Meat/Eggs)	Fish	Crustaceans	Mollusks
		Catfish	Crab	Abalone
Cow	Chicken	Cod	Crayfish	Clams
Goat	Duck	Flounder	Lobster	Mussels
Pig	Goose	Halibut	Prawn	Oysters
Rabbit	Hen	Mackerel	Shrimp	Scallops
Sheep	Turkey	Salmon		
		Sardine		
		Snapper		
		Trout		
		Tuna		

Table 4.4   Four-day Rotation Diet

Food Family	Food
Day 1	
Citrus	Lemon, orange, grapefruit, lime, tangerine, kumquat, citron
Banana	Banana, plantain, arrowroot (musa)
Palm	Coconut, date, date sugar
Parsley	Carrots, parsnips, celery, celery seed, celeriac, anise, dill, fennel, cumin, parsley, coriander, caraway
Spices	Black and white pepper, peppercorn, nutmeg, mace
Subucaya	Brazil nut
Birds	All fowl and game birds, including chicken, turkey, duck, goose, guinea, pigeon, quail, pheasant, eggs
Juices	Juices (preferably fresh) may be made and used from any fruits and vegetables listed above, in any combination desired, without adding sweeteners.
Day 2	
Grape	All varieties of grapes, raisins
Pineapple	Juice-pack, water-pack, or fresh
Rose	Strawberry, raspberry, blackberry, loganberry, rosehips
Gourds	Watermelon, cucumber, cantaloupe, pumpkin, squash, other melons, zucchini, pumpkin or squash seeds
Beet	Beet, spinach, chard
Legumes	Pea, black-eyed pea, dry beans, green beans, carob, soybeans, lentils, licorice, peanut, alfalfa
Cashew	Cashew, pistachio, mango
Birch	Filberts, hazelnuts
Flaxseed	Flaxseed
Swine	All pork products
Mollusks	Abalone, snail, squid, clam, mussel, oyster, scallop
Crustaceans	Crab, crayfish, lobster, prawn, shrimp
Juices	Juices (preferably fresh) may be made from any fruits, berries, or vegetables listed above and used without added sweeteners, in any combination desired, including fresh alfalfa and some legumes

Continued

Table 4.4   Four-day Rotation Diet *(continued)*

Food Family	Food
Day 3	
Apple	Apple, pear, quince
Gooseberry	Currant, gooseberry
Buckwheat	Buckwheat, rhubarb
Aster	Lettuce, chicory, endive, escarole, globe artichoke, dandelion, sunflower seeds, tarragon
Potato	Potato, tomato, eggplant, peppers (red and green), chili pepper, paprika, cayenne, ground cherries
Lily (onion)	Onion, garlic, asparagus, chives, beets
Spurge	Tapioca
Herb	Basil, savory, sage, oregano, horehound, catnip, spearmint, peppermint, thyme, marjoram, lemon balm
Walnut	English walnut, black walnut, pecan, hickory nut, butternut
Pedalium	Sesame
Beech	Chestnut
Saltwater fish	Herring, anchovy, cod, sea bass, sea trout, mackerel, tuna, swordfish, flounder, sole
Freshwater fish	Sturgeon, salmon, whitefish, bass, perch
Juices	Juices (preferably fresh) may be made from any fruits and vegetables listed above and used without added sweeteners, in any combination
Day 4	
Plums	Plum, cherry, peach, apricot, nectarine, almond, wild cherry
Blueberry	Blueberry, huckleberry, cranberry, wintergreen
Pawpaw	Pawpaw, papaya, papain
Mustard	Mustard, turnip, radish, horseradish, watercress, cabbage, Chinese cabbage, broccoli, cauliflower, brussels sprouts, kale, kohlrabi, rutabaga
Laurel	Avocado, cinnamon, bay leaf, sassafras, cassia buds or bark
Sweet potato or yam	
Grass	Wheat, corn, rice, oats, barley, rye, wild rice, cane, millet, sorghum, bamboo sprouts

Table 4.4 Four-day Rotation Diet *(continued)*

Food Family	Food
Orchid	Vanilla
Protea	Macadamia nut
Conifer	Pine nut
Fungus	Mushrooms and yeast (brewer's yeast, etc.)
Bovid	Milk products—butter, cheese, yogurt, beef and milk products, oleomargarine, lamb
Juices	Juices (preferably fresh) may be made from any fruits and vegetables listed above and used without added sweeteners, in any combination desired.

The Candida Control Diet

The dietary recommendations for controlling candida are straightforward: restrict your intake of refined carbohydrates, avoid milk and dairy products, avoid mold-containing foods, and identify and deal with food allergies. Below are concise recommendations of acceptable foods and foods to limit or avoid in the treatment of chronic candidiasis. (Note: foods to avoid because of either a high mold content or a tendency to raise blood sugar levels too quickly will be ~~stricken through~~.)

Vegetables

Vegetables provide the broadest range of nutrients of any food class. They are rich sources of vitamins, minerals, carbohydrates, and protein. The little fat they contain is in the form of essential fatty acids. Vegetables provide high quantities of other valuable health-promoting substances, especially fiber and carotenes. In Latin, the word *vegetable* means "to enliven or animate." Vegetables give us life.

Accumulated evidence shows that vegetables can prevent as well as treat many diseases.

Vegetables should play a major role in the diet. The U.S. National Academy of Science, the U.S. Department of Health and Human Services, and the National Cancer Institute recommend that Americans consume a minimum of three to five servings of vegetables per day.[17] Unfortunately, less than 11% of all Americans achieve this goal.

Vegetables are the richest sources of antioxidant compounds, which provide protection against free radicals. Free radicals are highly reactive molecules that can bind to and destroy cellular components. Free radicals have also been shown to be responsible for the initiation of many diseases including the two biggest killers of Americans—heart disease and cancer. Diabetics appear to be especially sensitive to the negative effects of free radicals. Increasing your intake of dietary antioxidants—such as carotenes, chlorophyll, vitamin C, sulfur-containing compounds, vitamin E, and selenium—by increasing the amounts of vegetables in your diet is essential in the long-term treatment of diabetes.

The best way to consume many vegetables is in their fresh, raw form. In their fresh form, many of the nutrients and health-promoting compounds of vegetables are provided in much higher concentrations. Drinking fresh vegetable juices is a phenomenal way to make sure that you are achieving your daily quota of vegetables.

When cooking vegetables it is very important that they not be overcooked. Overcooking will not only result in loss of important nutrients it will also alter the flavor of the vegetable. Light steaming, baking, and quick stir-frying are the best ways to cook vegetables. Do not boil vegetables unless you are making soup, because much of the nutrients would be left in the water. If fresh vegetables are not available, frozen vegetables are preferred to their canned counterparts.

Although pickled vegetables (such as pickles, sauerkraut, kim chee, etc.) are quite popular, they may not be healthful choices. Not only are they high in salt, they may also be high in cancer-causing compounds. Several population studies in China have suggested an association between consumption of pickled vegetables and cancer of the esophagus.[18] Pickled vegetables contain high concentrations of N-nitroso compounds. Once ingested, these compounds can form potent cancer-causing nitrosamines.

For those with chronic candidiasis, mushrooms, potatoes, winter squash, and yams should also be avoided.

Eat at least five servings of the following vegetables each day (note: serving size equals 2 cups raw and 1 cup cooked):

Artichoke

Asparagus

Bean sprouts

Beets

Broccoli

Brussels sprouts

Carrots

Cauliflower

Eggplant

Greens:

    Beet

    Chard

    Collard

    Dandelion

    Kale

    Mustard

    Spinach

    Turnip

~~Mushrooms~~

Okra

Onions

~~Parsnips~~

~~Potatoes~~

Rhubarb

Rutabaga

Sauerkraut

~~Squash, winter, acorn, or butternut~~

String beans, green or yellow

Summer squash

Tomatoes, tomato juice, vegetable juice cocktail

~~Yam~~

Zucchini

The following vegetables may be used as often as desired, especially in their raw form. In weight-loss programs, these vegetables are often referred to as "free foods" to be eaten in any desired amount because the calories they contain are offset by the number of calories that your body burns in the process of digesting them:

Alfalfa sprouts

Bell peppers

Bok choy

Cabbage

Chicory

Celery

Chinese cabbage

Cucumber

Endive

Escarole

Lettuce

Parsley

Radishes

Spinach

Turnips

Watercress

Grains

The important recommendation in regard to this food group is to choose whole grain products (e.g., whole grain breads, whole grain flour products, brown rice, etc.) over their processed counterparts (white bread, white flour products, white rice, etc.). Whole grains provide substantially more nutrients and health-promoting properties. Whole grains are a major source of complex carbohydrates, dietary fiber, minerals, and B vitamins. The protein content and quality of whole grains is greater than that of refined grains.

Diets rich in whole grains have been shown to be protective against the development of chronic degenerative diseases, especially cancer, heart disease, diabetes, varicose veins, and diseases of the colon including colon cancer, inflammatory bowel disease, hemorrhoids, and diverticulitis.[19] However, because most breads contain simple sugars in some form, I would recommend avoiding all breads until the candida is under control and then eating them only occasionally. Corn should also be avoided by those with candidiasis because of its high mold content. Choose five servings each day from the following list:

Whole grains (½ cup cooked)

Barley

Brown rice

~~Corn~~

Millet

Oats

Rice

Rye

Wheat

Legumes (Beans)

Legumes are among the oldest cultivated plants; fossil records demonstrate that even prehistoric people domesticated and cultivated certain legumes for food. Today, legumes are a mainstay in most diets of the world. Legumes are second only to grains in supplying calories and protein to the world's population. Compared to grains, they supply about the same number of total calories, but usually provide two to four times as much protein.

Legumes are often called the "poor people's meat," however, they might be better known as the "healthy people's meat." Although lacking some key amino acids, when legumes are combined with grains they form what is known as a *complete protein,* that is, a protein which contains sufficient levels of all the essential amino acids.

Legumes are fantastic foods because they are rich in important nutrients and health-promoting compounds. Legumes help to improve liver function, lower cholesterol levels, and are extremely effective in improving blood-sugar control.

Eat three servings (½ cup) of the following cooked or sprouted beans daily:

Black-eyed peas

Garbanzo beans

Kidney beans

Lentils

Lima beans

Pinto beans

Soybeans, including tofu

Split peas

Other dried beans and peas

Nuts and Seeds

Nuts and seeds are excellent nutritionally. They are especially good sources of essential fatty acids, vitamin E, protein, minerals, fiber, and other health-promoting substances. Because of the high oil content of nuts and seeds, one might suspect that the frequent consumption of nuts would increase the rate of obesity. But, in a large population study of 26,473 Americans, it was found that the people who consumed the most nuts were the least obese. This statistic is quite interesting. A possible explanation is that the nuts produced satiety, a feeling of appetite satisfaction. This same study also demonstrated that higher nut consumption was associated with a protective effect against heart attacks (both fatal and nonfatal).[20]

In general, nuts and seeds, due to their high oil content, are best purchased and stored in their shells. The shell is a natural protector against free radical damage caused by light and air. Make sure the shells are free from splits, cracks, stains, holes, or other surface imperfections. Do not eat or use moldy nuts or seeds; they are not safe. Also avoid limp, rubbery, dark, or shriveled nut meats. Store nuts and seeds with shells in a cool, dry environment. If whole, unshelled nuts and seeds are not available, make sure that the shelled nuts and seeds are stored in airtight containers in the refrigerator or freezer. Crushed, slivered, and chopped nuts are most often rancid. Prepare your own from the whole nut if a recipe calls for these. Try to have at least three servings of nuts and seeds per day. Peanuts and cashews should be avoided because of their high mold content.

Each of the following equals one serving:

Avocado (4-inch diameter), ⅛

Almonds, 8 whole

Brazil nuts, 2 large

~~Cashews~~

Filberts, 4 large

Flax seeds, 2 tablespoons

Hazelnuts, 4 large

Macadamia nuts, 5 medium

Olives, 5 small

Pecans, 2 large

~~Peanuts~~

Pine nuts, 2 tablespoons

Pistachios, 12 small

Pumpkin seeds, 2 tablespoons

Sesame seeds, 2 tablespoons

Sunflower seeds, 2 tablespoons

Walnuts, 6 small

About Fats

There are primarily two types of fats: saturated fats and unsaturated fats. Saturated fats are are typically animal fats and are solid at room temperature. In contrast, unsaturated fats (most vegetable oils) are liquid at room temperature. Our body requires two essential unsaturated fatty acids: linoleic acid and linolenic acid. These fatty acids function in our bodies as components of nerve cells, cellular membranes, and hormone-like substances known as *prostaglandins.* Increased consumption of essential fatty acids has been shown to lower cholesterol levels and improve many aspects of diabetes.

While essential fatty acids are critical to human health, too much fat in the diet, especially saturated fat, is linked to numerous cancers, heart disease, and strokes. It is strongly recommended by most nutritional experts that your total fat intake be kept below 30% of the total calories that you consume. It is also recommended that at least twice as much unsaturated fats be consumed as saturated fats. This recommendation is easy to follow by simply reducing the amount of animal products in your diet, increasing the amount of nuts and seeds consumed, and using natural polyunsaturated oils such as canola, olive, soy, and flaxseed oils as salad dressings.

Vegetable oils (serving size 1 tsp)
> Canola
>
> Corn
>
> Flaxseed
>
> Olive
>
> Safflower
>
> Soy
>
> Sunflower

Saturated Fats (avoid or use sparingly):
> Butter, 1 tsp
>
> Bacon, 1 slice
>
> ~~Cream, light or sour   2 tbsp~~
>
> ~~Cream, heavy   1 tbsp~~
>
> ~~Cream cheese   1 tbsp~~
>
> Salad dressings, 2 tsp
>
> Mayonnaise, 1 tsp

Milk and Other Dairy Products

As we discussed earlier this chapter, those with candidiasis should eliminate all milk and other dairy products from their diets. Dairy products are a common food allergen and contain substances that promote overgrowth of candida. Sometimes after resolution of symptoms, dairy foods can be reintroduced into the diet without problems. However, many people prone to chronic candidiasis may do better by eliminating these foods permanently.

Meats, Fish, and Eggs

When choosing foods from this list, it is important to choose primarily from the lowfat group and remove the skin of poultry, which will keep the amount of saturated fat low. Although many people advocate vegetarianism, the list below provides high concentrations of certain nutrients difficult to get in an entirely vegetarian diet, such as the full-range of amino acids, vitamin B_{12}, and iron.

Use these foods in small amounts as "condiments" in your diet rather than as mainstays. Keep portions small. Eat no more than four servings daily from this food group unless you are extremely physically active, in which case as many as eight servings per day may be consumed. Each of the following equals one serving:

Beef, 1 oz

Eggs, 1

Fish, 1 oz

Lamb, 1 oz

Poultry, 1 oz

Veal, 1 oz

Fruits

Fruits are a rich source of many beneficial compounds and regular fruit consumption has been shown to offer significant protection against many chronic degenerative diseases, including cancer, heart disease, cataracts, and strokes. Most individuals with chronic candidiasis can tolerate two to three servings of fruits per day, however, in severe cases, I recommend total exclusion until symptoms abate (typically within three months after beginning comprehensive therapy).

Each of the following equals one serving:

Fresh juice, 1 cup (8 oz)

Pasteurized juice, ⅔ cup

Apple, 1 large

Applesauce (unsweetened), 1 cup

Apricots (fresh), 4 medium

~~Apricots (dried), 8 halves~~

Banana, 1 medium

Berries

    Blackberries, 1 cup

    Blueberries, 1 cup

    Cranberries, 1 cup

    Raspberries, 1 cup

    Strawberries, 1½ cups

Cherries, 20 large

Dates, 4

Figs (fresh), 2

~~Figs (dried), 2~~

Grapefruit, 1

Grapes, 20

Mango, 1 small

~~Melons~~

   ~~Cantaloupe, ½ small~~

   ~~Honeydew, ¼ medium~~

   ~~Watermelon, 2 cups~~

Nectarines, 2 small

Orange, 1 large

Papaya, 1½ cups

Peaches, 2 medium

Persimmons, 2 medium

Pineapple, 1 cup

Plums, 4 medium

Prunes, 4 medium

Prune juice, ½ cup

~~Raisins, 4 tbsp~~

Tangerines, 2 medium

Final Comments

Following the straightforward dietary recommendations given in this chapter is absolutely essential in dealing with the yeast syndrome. Do not underestimate the importance of these recommendations. In fact, changing your diet may be the single most important step you take toward eliminating your candidiasis.[3]

5

Nutritional Supplementation

Nutritional supplementation is important for people with chronic candidiasis as well as for anyone wishing to achieve a higher level of wellness. Most of the patients that I see are placed on what I refer to as a *foundation* supplement program composed of a high-potency multiple vitamin and mineral supplement, extra antioxidants, and one tablespoon of flaxseed oil daily.

Taking a High-Quality Multiple Vitamin and Mineral Supplement

A high-quality multiple vitamin and mineral supplement that provides all of the known vitamins and minerals serves as a foundation upon which to build. Dr. Roger Williams, one of the premier biochemists of our time, states that healthy people should use multiple vitamin and mineral supplements as an "insurance formula" against possible deficiency. This does not mean that a deficiency will occur in the absence of the vitamin and mineral supplement, any more than not having fire insurance means that your house is going to burn down. But given the enormous potential for individual differences from person to person, and the varied mechanisms of vitamin and mineral actions, supplementation with a multiple formula makes sense especially when the nutrient-poor diet of most Americans is also considered.

For many key nutrients, my recommendations go well beyond the Recommended Dietary Allowances (RDAs) for vitamins and minerals, which are prepared by the Food and Nutrition Board of the National Research Council. These guidelines have been prepared periodically since 1941 and were originally developed to reduce the rates of diseases caused by severe nutritional deficiency, such as scurvy (deficiency of vitamin C), pellagra (deficiency of niacin), and beriberi (deficiency of vitamin B_1).

Another critical point is that the RDAs were designed to serve as the basis for evaluating the adequacy of diets of *groups* of people, not individuals. Individuals vary widely in their nutritional requirements and, as stated by the Food and Nutrition Board, "Individuals with special nutritional needs are not covered by the RDAs."[1]

A tremendous amount of scientific research indicates that the optimum level for many nutrients—especially the antioxidant nutrients vitamins C and E, beta-carotene, and selenium—may be much higher than their current RDAs. This is because the RDAs focus only on the *prevention* of nutritional deficiencies in population groups and do not define optimum intake for an individual.

Other factors that the RDAs do not adequately take into consideration are environmental and lifestyle factors, which can destroy vitamins and bind minerals. For example, even the Food and Nutrition Board acknowledges that smokers require at least twice as much vitamin C as nonsmokers do. But what about other nutrients and smoking?

And what about the effects of alcohol consumption, food additives, heavy metals (lead, mercury, etc.), carbon monoxide, and other chemicals associated with our modern society that are known to interfere with nutrient function? Dealing with the hazards of modern living is another reason why many people should take supplements.

While the RDAs have done a good job of defining nutrient intake levels to prevent nutritional deficiencies, there is still much to be learned regarding the optimum intake of nutrients. The recommendations in Tables 5.1 and 5.2 provide an optimum intake range in selecting a high-quality multiple vitamin and mineral supplement.

Taking Extra Antioxidants

The terms *antioxidants* and *free radicals* are becoming familiar to most health-minded individuals. Loosely defined, a free radical is a highly reactive molecule that can bind to and destroy body components. Free radical (oxidative) damage is what makes us age. Free radicals have been shown to be responsible for the initiation of many diseases including the two biggest killers of Americans—heart disease and cancer.

Antioxidants, in contrast, are compounds that help to protect against free radical damage. Antioxidant nutrients—such as beta-carotene, selenium, vitamin E, and vitamin C—have been shown to be very important in protecting against the development of heart disease, cancer, and other chronic degenerative diseases. In addition, antioxidants are thought to slow down the aging process.

Based on extensive data, it appears that a combination of antioxidants will provide greater antioxidant protection than any single nutritional antioxidant. Therefore, in addition to consuming a diet rich in plant foods, especially fruits and vegetables, I recommend using a combination

Table 5.1   Recommended Ranges for Supplemental Vitamins in International Units (IU), Milligrams (mg), or Micrograms (mcg)

Vitamin	Range for Adults
Vitamin A (retinol)	2,500 IU
Note: Women of child-bearing age should not take more than 2,500 IU of retinol daily due to the possible risk of birth defects if becoming pregnant is a possibility.	
Vitamin A (from beta-carotene)	5,000–25,000 IU
Vitamin D	100–400 IU
Note: Elderly people in nursing homes living in northern latitudes should supplement at the high range.	
Vitamin E (d-alpha tocopherol)	400–800 IU
Note: It may be more cost-effective to take vitamin E separately.	
Vitamin K (phytonadione)	60–300 mcg
Vitamin C (ascorbic acid)	500–1,500 mg
Note: It may be easier to take vitamin C separately.	
Vitamin B_1 (thiamin)	10–100 mg
Vitamin B_2 (riboflavin)	10–50 mg
Niacin	10–100 mg
Niacinamide	10–30 mg
Vitamin B_6 (pyridoxine)	25–150 mg
Biotin	100–300 mcg
Pantothenic acid	25–100 mg
Folic acid	400 mcg
Vitamin B_{12}	400 mcg
Choline	10–100 mg
Inositol	10–100 mg

of antioxidant nutrients rather than high dosages of any single antioxidant. Mixtures of antioxidant nutrients work together harmoniously to produce the phenomena of synergy, where the total effect is greater than the sum of the individual elements.

The two primary antioxidants in the human body are vitamin C and vitamin E. Vitamin C is an *aqueous-phase*

Table 5.2 Recommended Ranges for Supplemental Minerals in Milligrams (mg) or Micrograms (mcg)

Mineral	Range for Adults
Boron	1–6 mg
Calcium	250–1,250 mg

Note: Taking a separate calcium supplement may be necessary when trying to achieve higher dosage levels in women at risk for or suffering from osteoporosis.

Chromium	200–400 mcg

Note: For diabetes and weight loss, dosages of 600 mcg can be used.

Copper	1–2 mg
Iodine	50–150 mcg
Iron	15–30 mg

Note: Men and postmenopausal women rarely need supplemental iron.

Magnesium	250–500 mg

Note: When magnesium therapy is indicated, take a separate magnesium supplement.

Manganese	10–15 mg
Molybdenum	10–25 mcg
Potassium	200–500 mg
Selenium	100–200 mcg
Silica	1–25 mg
Vanadium	50–100 mcg
Zinc	15–45 mg

antioxidant, which means that it is found in body compartments composed of water. In contrast, vitamin E is a *lipid-phase* antioxidant because it is found in lipid-soluble body compartments such as cell membranes and fatty molecules.

If you are taking a high-potency multiple vitamin and mineral formula, many of the supportive antioxidant nutrients, such as selenium, zinc, and beta-carotene, are provided for. Therefore, your primary concern may be simply to ensure beneficial levels of vitamin C and vitamin E. Below are my daily supplementation guidelines for these key nutritional antioxidants for supporting general health. Be sure to check how much your multiple vitamin and mineral formula is providing.

Vitamin E (d-alpha tocopherol)	400 to 800 IU
Vitamin C (ascorbic acid)	500 to 1,500 mg

Taking One Tablespoon of Flaxseed Oil Daily

In this day and age of concern over fat in your food, a recommendation to supplement your daily diet with one tablespoon of flaxseed oil may be puzzling. However, as you'll discover, this recommendation makes perfectly good sense. While it is true you should not consume more than 30% of your daily calories as fats, a lack of the dietary essential fatty acids has been suggested as playing a significant role in the development of many chronic degenerative diseases, including heart disease, cancer, and strokes.

It is estimated by many experts that approximately 80% of Americans consume an insufficient quantity of essential fatty acids. This dietary insufficiency presents a serious health threat. In addition to providing the body with energy, the essential fatty acids function in our bodies as components of nerve cells, cellular membranes, and hormone-like substances known as prostaglandins.

As well as playing a critical role in normal physiology, essential fatty acids are protective and therapeutic against heart disease, cancer, auto-immune diseases such as multiple sclerosis and rheumatoid arthritis, skin diseases, and many others. Over 60 health conditions have been shown to benefit from essential fatty acid supplementation.[2]

Organic, unrefined flaxseed oil is considered by many to be the answer to restoring the body's proper level of essential fatty acids. Flaxseed oil is unique because it contains both essential fatty acids: alpha linolenic (an omega-3 fatty acid) and linoleic acid (an omega-6 fatty acid) in appreciable amounts. Flaxseed oil is the world's richest source of omega-3 fatty acids; it contains more than two times the amount of omega-3 fatty acids than fish oils do.

Final Comments

A deficiency of any of a number of nutrients can lead to impaired immune function or poor detoxification processes, which could result in an overgrowth of *Candida albicans*. Numerous studies have shown that nutrient deficiency is quite common in patients with *Candida albicans* infections.[3,4] The recommendations in this chapter go a long way toward addressing some of our goals in the treatment of candidiasis, such as enhancing immune and liver function, by providing your body with the building blocks that it needs.

6

Enhancing Immunity

Recurrent or chronic infections, including chronic candidiasis, are characterized by a depressed immune system. A vicious cycle makes it difficult for people with depressed immune systems to overcome chronic candidiasis: A compromised immune system leads to infection and infection leads to damage to the immune system, further weakening resistance.

Too often the importance of susceptibility to infection or disease is overlooked by conventional medicine (see Chapter 2). Support and enhancement of immune-system function is an absolute must if you have chronic candidiasis.

What Is the Immune System?

The immune system is one of the most complex and fascinating systems of the human body. The immune system's primary function is protecting the body against infection and the development of cancer.

The immune system is composed of the lymphatic vessels and organs (thymus, spleen, tonsils, and lymph nodes), white blood cells (lymphocytes, neutrophils, basophils, eosinophils, monocytes, etc.), specialized cells residing in various tissues (macrophages, mast cells, etc.), and specialized serum factors.

The Thymus

The thymus is the major gland of the immune system. It is composed of two soft pinkish-gray lobes lying in a bib-like fashion just below the thyroid gland and above the heart. To a very large extent, the health of the thymus determines the health of the immune system. Individuals who get frequent infections or suffer from chronic infections typically have impaired thymus activity. Also, people affected with hay fever, allergies, migraine headaches, and rheumatoid arthritis usually have altered thymus function.

The thymus is responsible for many immune-system functions, including the production of T lymphocytes, a type of white blood cell responsible for *cell-mediated immunity.* Cell-mediated immunity refers to immune mechanisms not controlled or mediated by antibodies.

Cell-mediated immunity is extremely important in the resistance of the body to *Candida albicans.* It is also extremely important in protecting against infections caused by viruses (including Herpes simplex, Epstein-Barr, and the viruses that cause hepatitis) and mold-like bacteria such as *Chlamydia.* Finally, cell-mediated immunity is critical in protecting against the development of cancer, auto-immune disorders such as rheumatoid arthritis, and allergies.

The thymus gland releases several hormones, such as thymosin, thymopoeitin, and serum thymic factor, which regulate many immune functions. Low levels of these hormones in the blood are associated with depressed immunity and an increased susceptibility to infection. Typically, thymic hormone levels are very low in the elderly, individuals prone to infection, cancer and AIDS patients, and individuals exposed to undue stress.

Lymph, Lymphatic Vessels, and Lymph Nodes

Approximately one-sixth of the entire body is composed of the space between cells. Collectively this space is referred to as the *interstitium* and the fluid contained within this space is referred to as the *interstitial fluid.* This fluid flows into the lymphatic vessels and becomes lymph.

Lymphatic vessels usually run parallel to arteries and veins. The vessels function in draining waste products from tissues. The lymphatic vessels transport the lymph to lymph nodes, which filter the lymph. The cells responsible for this filtering are macrophages. These large cells engulf and destroy foreign particles, including bacteria and cellular debris.

The lymph nodes also contain B-lymphocytes, the white blood cells that are capable of initiating antibody production in response to the presence of viruses, bacteria, yeast, and other organisms.

The Spleen

The spleen is the largest mass of lymphatic tissue in the body. Weighing about 7 ounces, the spleen is a fist-sized, spongy, dark-purple organ that lies in the upper left abdomen behind the lower ribs. The spleen's functions include producing white blood cells, engulfing and destroying bacteria and cellular debris, and destroying worn-out red blood cells and platelets. The spleen also serves as a blood reservoir. During times of demand, such as hemorrhage, the spleen can release its stored blood and prevent shock.

Like the thymus, the spleen also releases many potent immune-system enhancing compounds. For example, tuft-sin and splenopentin, two small peptides secreted by the spleen, as well as spleen extracts, have been shown to exert profound immune-enhancing activity.[1-4]

White Blood Cells

There are several types of white blood cells including neutrophils, eosinophils, basophils, lymphocytes, and monocytes.

Neutrophils   These cells actively phagocytize (engulf and destroy) bacteria, tumor cells, and dead particulate matter. Neutrophils are especially important in preventing bacterial infection.

Eosinophils and Basophils   These cells secrete histamine and other compounds, which are designed to break down antigen–antibody complexes, but which also promote allergic mechanisms.

T-Cells   T-cells stand for *thymus-derived lymphocytes.* These cells orchestrate many immune functions and are the major components of cell-mediated immunity (discussed above). The different types of T-cells include helper T-cells, which help other white blood cells to function; suppressor T-cells, which inhibit white blood cell functions; and cytotoxic T-cells, which attack and destroy foreign tissue, cancer cells, and virus-infected cells.

T-Cell Ratios   The ratio of helper T-cells to suppressor T-cells is a useful determinant of immune function. If the ratio is low, immunodeficiency is present. For example, AIDS is characterized by a very low ratio of helper T-cells to suppressor T-cells. If the ratio of helper T-cells to suppressor T-cells is high, most often allergies or autoimmune disorders such as rheumatoid arthritis and lupus are present.

B Cells B cells are responsible for producing antibodies, which are large protein molecules that bind to foreign molecules (antigens) on bacteria, viruses, other organisms, and tumor cells. After the antibody binds to the antigen, it sets up a sequence of events that ultimately destroys the infectious organism or tumor cell.

Natural Killer Cells Natural killer cells (NK cells) received their name because of their ability to destroy cells that have become cancerous or infected with viruses. They are the body's first line of defense against cancer development. The level or activity of natural killer cells is typically low in patients with chronic fatigue syndrome.

Monocytes Monocytes are the garbage collectors of the body. These large white blood cells are responsible for cleaning up cellular debris after an infection. Monocytes are also responsible for triggering many immune responses.

Special Tissue Cells

There are two specialized white blood cells that reside in tissues—macrophages and mast cells.

Macrophages As stated earlier, the lymph is filtered by specialized cells known as macrophages. Macrophages are actually monocytes that have taken up residence in specific tissues such as the liver, spleen, and lymph nodes. These large cells engulf foreign particles, including bacteria and cellular debris. Macrophages are essential in protecting against invasion by microorganisms as well as against damage to the lymphatic system.

Mast cells Mast cells are basophils that have taken up residence primarily along blood vessels. The mast cell, like the basophil, is responsible for releasing histamine and other compounds involved in allergic reactions.

Special Chemical Factors

A number of special chemical factors enhance the immune system (interferon, interleukin II, complement fractions, etc.). These compounds are produced by various white blood cells. For example, interferon is produced primarily by T-cells, interleukins are produced by macrophages and T-cells, and complement fractions are manufactured in the liver and spleen. These special chemical factors are extremely important in activating the white blood cells that destroy cancer cells and viruses.

Immune Function and Chronic Candidiasis

The importance of a healthy immune system in protecting against candida overgrowth is well-known by any physician who has seen a patient suffering from AIDS or taking drugs that suppress the immune system. In either case, severe overgrowth of *Candida albicans* is a hallmark feature, one which provides considerable evidence that attaining better immune function is absolutely essential in patients with chronic candidiasis.

In addition, in my clinical practice, I have found that my patients with chronic candidiasis often suffer from other chronic infections, presumably due to a depressed immune system. Typically this depression of immune function is related to decreased thymus function manifesting primarily as depressed cell-mediated immunity. Although I do not perform expensive laboratory tests to document this depression, I believe it to exist based upon these patients' histories of repeated viral infections (including the common cold), frequent outbreaks of cold sores or genital herpes, and prostatic (men) or vaginal (women) infections.

Causes of Depressed Immune Function in Candidiasis

As I've said before, the patient with chronic candidiasis is typically stuck in a vicious cycle. A triggering event such as antibiotic use or nutrient deficiency can lead to immune suppression, thus allowing *Candida albicans* to overgrow and become more firmly entrenched in the lining of the gastrointestinal tract. (See Table 6.1.) Once the organism attaches itself to the intestinal cells, it competes with the cells and ultimately the entire body for nutrients—robbing the body of vital nutrition.

In addition, *Candida albicans* secretes a large number of toxins (known as mycotoxins) and antigens (substances that promote an immune response).[5,6] *Candida albicans* is referred to as a *polyantigenic* organism because over 79 distinct antigens have been identified. Because of the tremendous number of antigens, an overgrowth of *Candida albicans* greatly taxes the immune system. Thus, restoring proper immune function is one of the key goals in the treatment of chronic candidiasis.

Restoring Proper Immune Function

There isn't any single magic bullet that can immediately restore immune function in patients with chronic candidiasis. Instead, a comprehensive approach involving lifestyle changes, stress management, exercise, diet, nutritional supplementation, glandular therapy, and the use of plant-based medicines should be used.

Table 6.1   Triggers to Impaired Immunity in Candidiasis

Antibiotic use

Corticosteroid use

Other drugs that suppress the immune system (e.g., chemotherapy drugs, plaquinil, and methotrexate)

Nutrient deficiencies

Food allergies

High-sugar diet

Stress

The Influence of Mood and Attitude on Immune Function

The overall function of the immune system is intricately tied to mood and attitude. Simplistically speaking, when we are happy and upbeat, our immune system functions much better. Conversely, when we are depressed, our immune system tends to be depressed. Many of the patients that I have seen with chronic candidiasis are understandably depressed and frustrated by their condition. However, it is absolutely critical to focus on the positive aspects of life and to learn to laugh often in order to achieve optimum function of the immune system.

The healing power of laughter was highlighted in Norman Cousins's popular book *Anatomy of an Illness*.[7] This book caused a significant stir in the medical community when it was published in 1979. Cousins provided an autobiographical account of his attempts to fight a serious disease, which showed that laughter and positive emotional states can help heal the body. Cousins watched the TV show "Candid Camera" and Marx brothers' films and read humorous books.

Originally physicians and researchers scoffed at Cousins's account. However, numerous studies have demonstrated that laughter and other positive emotional states can, in fact, enhance the immune system.[8,9]

By laughing frequently and taking a lighter view of life, you will find that life is much more enjoyable and fun. Here are eight tips to help you inject more laughter into your life.

1. Learn to laugh at yourself.
2. Inject humor whenever it is appropriate.
3. Read the comics in order to find a comic that you find funny and follow it.
4. Watch comedies on television.
5. Go to comedies at the movie theater.
6. Listen to comedy audiotapes in your car while commuting.
7. Play with kids.
8. Ask yourself the question: "What is funny about this situation?"

Stress and the Immune System

Stress can be one of the triggering events that leads to depression of the immune system and the overgrowth and entrenchment of *Candida albicans* in the gastrointestinal or vaginal tract. Stress causes increases in the output of adrenal gland hormones, including adrenaline and corticosteroids. Among other things, these hormones inhibit white blood cells and cause the thymus gland to shrink. High levels of these hormones circulating in the blood lead to a significant suppression of immune function, leaving the body susceptible to infections, cancer, and other illnesses. The level of immune suppression is usually proportional to the level of stress.[10,11]

Stress results in stimulation of the sympathetic nervous system, which is responsible for the fight-or-flight response. The immune system functions better under the parasympathetic nervous system.[12] This portion of our autonomic nervous system assumes control over bodily functions during periods of rest, relaxation, visualization, meditation, and sleep. For example during the deepest levels of sleep, potent immune-enhancing compounds are released and many immune functions are greatly increased.[13]

The value of quality sleep and relaxation techniques for counteracting the effects of stress and enhancing our immune system cannot be overemphasized. Here are ten tips to help deal with stress and enhance immune function:

1. Don't starve your emotional life. Foster meaningful relationships. Provide time to give and receive love in your life.

2. Learn to be a good listener. Allow the people in your life to share their feelings and thoughts with you without interrupting. Empathize with them, put yourself in their shoes.

3. Don't try to talk over somebody. If you find yourself being interrupted, relax, don't try to outtalk the other person. If you are courteous and allow them to speak, eventually (unless they are extremely rude) they will respond in kind. If they don't, point out to them that they are interrupting the communication process. You can only do this if you have been a good listener.

4. Avoid aggressive or passive behavior. Be assertive, but express your thoughts and feelings in a kind way to help improve relationships at work and at home.

5. Avoid excessive stress in your life as best you can by avoiding excessive work hours, poor nutrition, and inadequate rest. Get as much sleep as you can.

6. Avoid stimulants such as caffeine and nicotine. Stimulants promote the fight-or-flight response and tend to make people more irritable.

7. Take time to build long-term health and success by performing stress-reduction techniques and deep breathing exercises.

8. Accept gracefully those things over which you have no control. Save your energy for those things that you can do something about.

9. Accept yourself. Remember that you are human and will make mistakes along the way to learn from.

10. Be more patient and tolerant of other people. Follow the Golden Rule.

The Influence of Lifestyle on Immune Function

A healthful lifestyle goes a long way toward establishing a healthy immune system. Of particular interest to individuals with chronic candidiasis are the results from several studies that have examined the effect of lifestyle on immune function.[14,15] The following practices were associated with a higher level of immune function:

1. Not smoking
2. Increased intake of green vegetables
3. Regular meals
4. Proper body weight
5. More than seven hours of sleep per night

6. Regular exercise
7. A vegetarian diet

Diet and Immune Function

The health of the immune system is largely determined by the body's state of stress and nutritional status. Dietary factors that depress immune function include nutrient deficiency, sugar, and high cholesterol levels. Dietary factors that enhance immune function include all the essential nutrients, antioxidants, carotenes, and flavonoids.

Consistent with good health, optimum immune function requires a healthful diet that (1) is rich in whole, natural foods, such as fruits, vegetables, grains, beans, seeds, and nuts; (2) is low in fats and refined sugars; (3) contains adequate, but not excessive, amounts of protein; and (4) includes drinking five to six 8-ounce glasses of water per day.

These dietary recommendations, along with a positive mental attitude, a high-potency multivitamin-mineral supplement, a regular exercise program of at least 30 minutes of aerobic exercise four times per week, daily deep breathing and relaxation exercises (meditation, prayer, etc.), and at least seven hours of sleep daily will go a long way toward helping the immune system function at an optimum level.

Let's take a closer look at some of the specific dietary factors that can play a role in immune function.

Poor Diet Resulting in Nutrient Deficiency

Nutrient deficiency is the most frequent cause of a depressed immune system. Nutrition surveys of the U.S. population have shown that most Americans are deficient in at least one nutrient.[16] And, as stated in the last chapter, numerous studies also have shown that patients with chronic candidiasis have a higher frequency of nutrient deficiency than healthy subjects.[17,18] The significance of these findings is substantial because virtually any nutrient deficiency will result in an impaired immune system, making an individual predisposed to chronic infections as well as an increased risk for cancer. The recommendations in Chapters 4 and 5 go a long way toward ensuring optimal intake of nutrients.

Obesity and Elevated Fats in the Blood

Americans are typically overfed, but undernourished. The nutritional deficiencies and the nutritional excesses team up to greatly reduce immune function. Obesity is not only associated with such conditions as atherosclerosis, hypertension, diabetes mellitus, and joint disorders, it is also associated with decreased immune status, as evidenced by the decreased bacteria-killing activity of neutrophils, as well as increased morbidity and mortality from infections and cancer.[19]

Because cholesterol and fat levels in the blood are usually elevated in obese individuals, this may explain their impaired immune function. Increased blood levels of cholesterol, free fatty acids, triglycerides, and bile acids inhibit various immune functions.[19] Therefore optimum immune function is dependent on maintaining healthy levels of cholesterol and other fats in the blood.

Sugar

The high-sugar diet of many Americans may be contributing to a state of immune suppression and increased susceptibility to chronic candidiasis. Ingestion of sugar has been shown to adversely affect the immune system.[20-22] Considering that the average American consumes 150 grams of sucrose, plus other refined simple sugars, each day, the inescapable conclusion is that most Americans have chronically depressed immune systems. Sugar is also the primary fuel for *Candida albicans.* It is crystal clear that individuals with chronic candidiasis must absolutely avoid refined sugar.

Enhancing Thymus Gland Activity

Perhaps the most effective method for reestablishing a healthy immune system is employing measures designed to improve thymus function. Promoting optimum thymus gland activity involves:

1. Preventing thymic involution (shrinkage) by ensuring adequate dietary intake of antioxidant nutrients such as carotenes, vitamin C, vitamin E, zinc, and selenium
2. Consuming nutrients that are required in the manufacture or action of thymic hormones
3. Using products containing concentrates of calf thymus tissue

Antioxidants and Thymus Function

The thymus gland shows maximum development immediately after birth. During the aging process the thymus gland undergoes a process of involution (shrinkage). The reason for this involution is that the thymus gland is extremely susceptible to free radical and oxidative damage caused by stress, radiation, infection, and chronic illness.

It is thought that individuals with chronic candidiasis suffer from a state of oxidative imbalance. In other words, these patients have a greater number of pro-oxidants in their system than antioxidants. It is important to supplement the diet with antioxidants such as vitamin C, vitamin E, selenium, zinc, and beta-carotene according to the guidelines given in Chapter 5. These nutrients have been shown to prevent thymic involution and enhance cell-mediated immune functions.[23-25]

Nutrients Required for Thymic Hormone Manufacture or Action

Many nutrients function as important cofactors in the manufacture, secretion, and function of thymic hormones. Deficiencies in any one of these nutrients result in decreased thymic hormone action and impaired immune function. Zinc, vitamin B_6, and vitamin C are perhaps the most critical nutrients. Supplementation with these nutrients increases thymic hormone function and cell-mediated immunity.[26,27] Again, following the guidelines in Chapter 5 will provide optimum levels of these important nutrients.

Correcting a Zinc Deficiency Zinc is probably the most critical nutrient involved in thymus gland function and thymus hormone action. Zinc is involved in virtually every aspect of immunity. When zinc levels are low, the number of T-cells is reduced, thymic hormone levels are lower, and many white blood functions critical to the immune response are severely lacking. All of these effects are reversible upon adequate zinc administration.[26,27] Not surprisingly, low zinc levels have been found in women suffering from recurrent vaginal candida infections.[28]

The dosage range for zinc supplementation for general health support is 15 to 20 mg daily. Since the average American consumes about 10 mg of zinc per day, supplementing with an additional 15 to 20 mg results in a daily intake of 25 to 30 mg for most people. There are many forms of zinc to choose from. Zinc bound to picolinate, acetate, citrate, glycerate, or monomethionine are all excellent forms of zinc.

Enhancing Thymus Function with Thymus Extracts

A substantial amount of clinical data supports the effectiveness of orally administered calf-thymus extracts in restoring and enhancing immune function.[29,30] One of the basic concepts of glandular therapy is that the oral ingestion of glandular material of a particular animal gland will strengthen the corresponding human gland. Thymus extract acts as a broad-spectrum immune-system enhancer, which is presumably a result of improved thymus gland activity.

The appropriate dosage will vary from one manufacturer to another because there are no quality-control procedures or standards enforced in the glandular extracts industry; it is up to the individual companies to adopt quality control and good manufacturing procedures.

From a practical view, products concentrated and standardized for polypeptide content are preferable to crude preparations. In my practice I recommend Thymulus (a product of Enzymatic Therapy), which is a high-quality thymus extract concentrated for polypeptide content. A good daily dosage when using this or similar products is two capsules daily to provide 750 mg of crude polypeptide fractions. No side effects or adverse effects have been reported with the use of thymus preparations.

Plant-Based Medicines

Many herbs have shown remarkable effects in enhancing and modulating immune functions. Modern research is verifying what herbal practitioners have known for thousands of years: Herbs work with our bodily systems to promote health. Chapter 9 details some of the more popular plant-based medicines that can be utilized to enhance the immune system and fight candida overgrowth.

Final Comments

This chapter has detailed the immune system, its various components, and natural ways to enhance its function. Perhaps the most important determinant of immune status is lifestyle. Maintaining a positive attitude, adopting a healthful lifestyle, dealing with stress, following the dietary guidelines, and ensuring optimum levels of essential nutrients and antioxidants are critical to a healthy immune system. To provide additional support, preparations containing calf-thymus tissue can be extremely helpful in restoring healthy immune system function in patients with chronic candidiasis.

7

Promoting Detoxification

Candida patients usually exhibit multiple chemical sensitivities and allergies, indicators that their detoxification reactions are stressed. Therefore, candida patients need to support liver function. In fact, improving the health of the liver and promoting detoxification is a critical factor in the successful treatment of candidiasis.

The Importance of the Liver

To a very large extent, the health, vitality, and energy levels of an individual are determined by the health and vitality of the liver. The liver is truly an intricate, complex, and remarkable organ. It is, without question, the most important organ of metabolism.

The liver is the organ that deals with the constant onslaught of toxic chemicals from the body and environment. Toxic chemicals from the environment are everywhere—in the air that we breathe and the water and food that we consume. Some of the toxic chemicals known to pass through the liver include heavy metals such as lead, cadmium, mercury, and aluminum; solvents such as formaldehyde, toluene, and acetone; the polycyclic hydrocarbons, which are components of various herbicides and pesticides, including DDT, dioxin, 2,4,5-T, 2,4-D; and the halogenated compounds PCB and PCP. Although our exact degree of exposure to these compounds is not known, it is probably quite high; yearly production of synthetic pesticides exceeds 1.4 billion pounds in the United States alone and the United States alone also dumps over 600,000 tons of lead into the atmosphere each year.[1,2]

Detoxification of harmful substances is a continuous process in the body. The ability to detoxify and eliminate toxins largely determines an individual's health status, including the status of the immune system.

The Liver and Immune Function

The health and function of the liver is critically linked to the status of the immune system. Although not technically considered an organ of the immune system, the liver plays a role in a variety of functions essential to a healthy immune system. Specifically, the liver produces physiological substances required by the immune system (e.g., complement, a specialized system composed of serum factors that ultimately destroy microorganisms, cancer cells, and foreign material). The liver also is the major producer of lymph in the body and, with the help of special white blood cells known as Kupffer cells, is responsible for filtering the blood and removing cellular debris, bacteria, viruses, yeast, and toxic foreign compounds that have been absorbed by the gastrointestinal tract. Kupffer cells, when functioning properly, can engulf and destroy a single bacteria in less than $\frac{1}{100}$ second.

Damage to the Liver and Chronic Candidiasis

Damage to the liver is often an underlying factor in chronic candidiasis as well as in chronic fatigue syndrome. When the liver is even slightly damaged by chemical toxins, immune function is severely compromised.

The effect of nonviral liver damage on suppressing the immune system has been repeatedly demonstrated in experimental animal studies and human studies. For example, when the liver of a rat has been damaged by a chemical toxin, immune function is severely hindered.[3] Liver injury is also linked to candida overgrowth as is evident from studies of mice, which demonstrate that when the liver is even slightly damaged, candida runs rampant through the body.[4]

The classic human example of the effect of liver injury on immune function is seen with alcohol ingestion. This is most evident in the alcoholic, but ingestion of as little as 1 to 2 ounces of alcohol is enough to induce injury and lead to immune suppression in some individuals. The levels of antioxidant nutrients such as vitamin C, vitamin E, selenium, and zinc appear to be critical factors in determining the extent of the immune-system impairment after alcohol ingestion.

Antioxidants are essential to protect the liver from damage. Optimum tissue concentrations of these compounds should be maintained in order to support liver health. The guidelines in Chapter 5 provide a strong foundation for optimum concentrations of these antioxidants.

Supporting the Liver

A rational approach to aiding the body's detoxification involves: (1) eating a diet that focuses on fresh fruits and vegetables, whole grains, legumes, nuts, and seeds;

(2) adopting a healthful lifestyle, including avoiding alcohol and exercising regularly; (3) taking a high-potency multiple vitamin and mineral supplement; (4) using special nutritional and herbal supplements to protect the liver and enhance liver function; and (5) going on a three-day fast at the change of each season (or four times a year).

Diet and Liver Function

The first step toward supporting proper liver function is following the dietary recommendations given in Chapter 4. Such a diet will provide a wide range of essential nutrients, which the liver needs to carry out its important functions. If you want to have a healthy liver, stay away from: (1) saturated fats, (2) refined sugar, and (3) alcohol.

Special foods rich in factors that help to protect the liver from damage and improve liver function include foods high in sulfur such as garlic, legumes, onions, and eggs; good sources of water-soluble fibers such as pears, oat bran, apples, and legumes; cabbage-family vegetables, especially broccoli, brussels sprouts, and cabbage; artichokes, beets, carrots, and dandelions; and many herbs and spices such as turmeric, cinnamon, and licorice.

Lifestyle Changes

Lifestyle goes a long way toward promoting detoxification. Reduce your toxic load by avoiding such detrimental habits as excessive alcohol consumption and exposure to cigarette smoke. Regular aerobic exercise also helps by promoting improved lymphatic flow and immune function.

Avoid Alcohol   Alcohol stresses detoxification processes and can lead to liver damage and immune suppression. If you suffer from chronic candidiasis, I recommend that you eliminate consumption of alcohol entirely. After you have regained your vigor, if you are going to drink, limit your intake to no more than one drink per day and be sure to employ all the other measures discussed in this chapter to support your liver.

Supplement with Vitamins and Minerals   A high-potency multiple vitamin and mineral supplement is a must for dealing with the toxic chemicals that we are constantly exposed to. Antioxidants such as vitamin C, beta-carotene, and vitamin E are quite important in protecting the liver from damage as well as helping in detoxification mechanisms. However, even simple nutrients such as the B vitamins, calcium, and trace minerals are critical to the elimination of heavy metals and other toxic compounds from the body.[5–7]

Additional Liver Support

For most individuals suffering from chronic candidiasis, following the dietary recommendations given in Chapter 4 and the recommendations for nutritional supplementation in Chapter 5 will provide all the support they need to improve liver function. However, in cases where liver function is not quite up to par I recommend taking special nutritional and herbal factors as well as going on a three-day fast.

How do you determine if your liver is working properly? There are some special tests that can determine liver function, but I recommend simply looking over the following list. If any factor applies to you, take the lipotropic agents and the silymarin (both described below).

Indications of Impaired Liver Function

More than 20 pounds overweight

Diabetes

Presence of gallstones

History of heavy alcohol use

    Psoriasis
    Natural and synthetic steroid hormone use:
        Anabolic steroids
        Estrogens
        Oral contraceptives
    High exposure to certain chemicals or drugs:
        Cleaning solvents
        Pesticides
        Antibiotics
        Diuretics
        Nonsteroidal anti-inflammatory drugs
    Synthroid or other thyroid hormone medication
    History of viral hepatitis

Lipotropic Agents The nutrients choline, betaine, and methionine are referred to as *lipotropic agents*. Lipotropic agents are compounds that promote the flow of fat and bile to and from the liver. In essence, they produce a "decongestant" effect on the liver and promote improved liver function and fat metabolism.

Formulas containing lipotropic agents are very useful in enhancing detoxification reactions and other liver functions. Lipotropic formulas have been used to treat a wide variety of conditions by nutrition-oriented physicians, including a number of liver disorders such as hepatitis, cirrhosis, and chemical-induced liver disease.

Most major manufacturers of nutritional supplements offer lipotropic formulas. When taking a lipotropic formula, be sure to take enough of the formula to provide a daily dose of 1,000 mg of choline and 1,000 mg of either methionine and/or cysteine.

Lipotropic formulas appear to increase the levels of two important liver substances: SAM (S-adenosylmethionine), the major lipotropic compound in the liver, and glutathione, one of the major detoxifying compounds in the liver.[8-10]

Silymarin Many plants exert beneficial effects on liver function. However, the most impressive results have been produced by a special extract of milk thistle (*Silybum marianum*) known as silymarin. Silymarin refers to a group of flavonoid compounds, which exert tremendous effect on protecting the liver from damage as well as enhancing detoxification processes.

Silymarin prevents damage to the liver by acting as an antioxidant and is many times more potent in antioxidant activity than vitamins E and C.[11-13] The protective effect of silymarin against liver damage has been demonstrated by a number of experimental studies. Experimental liver damage in animals is produced by extremely toxic chemicals such as carbon tetrachloride, amanita toxin, galactosamine, and praseodymium nitrate. Silymarin has been shown to protect against liver damage by all of these agents.[11-13]

One of the key ways in which silymarin enhances detoxification reactions is by preventing the depletion of glutathione. The level of glutathione in the liver is critically linked to the liver's ability to detoxify. That is, the higher the glutathione content, the greater the liver's capacity to detoxify harmful chemicals. Typically, when we are exposed to chemicals (including alcohol) that damage the liver, the concentration of glutathione is substantially reduced. This reduction in glutathione makes the liver's cells susceptible to damage. Silymarin not only prevents the depletion of glutathione induced by alcohol and other toxic chemicals, but has been shown to increase the level of glutathione in the liver by up to 35%.[14] Since the ability of the liver to detoxify is largely related to its level of glutathione, the results seem to indicate that silymarin can increase detoxification reactions by up to 35%.

In human studies, silymarin has been shown to have positive effects in treating liver diseases of various kinds, including cirrhosis, chronic hepatitis, fatty infiltration of the liver (chemical- and alcohol-induced fatty liver), and inflammation of the bile duct.[15-19]

Silymarin products are available at health food stores. The standard dosage for silymarin is 70 to 210 mg three times daily. (Note: higher dosages are more effective than lower dosages in cases of definite liver disorders.) Continue taking silymarin for a minimum of one month or until a resolution of elevated liver enzymes occurs as demonstrated by a blood analysis.

Fasting

Fasting is often used as a detoxification method because it is one of the quickest ways to increase elimination of wastes and enhance the healing processes of the body. Fasting is defined as abstinence from all food and drink except water for a specific period of time, usually for a therapeutic or religious purpose.

Although fasting is probably one of the oldest known therapies, it has been largely ignored by the conventional medical community despite the fact that significant scientific research on the benefits of fasting exists. Numerous medical journals have carried articles on the use of fasting in the treatment of obesity, chemical poisoning, rheumatoid arthritis, allergies, psoriasis, eczema, thrombophlebitis, leg ulcers, irritable bowel syndrome, impaired or deranged appetite, bronchial asthma, depression, neurosis, and schizophrenia.

One of the most significant studies regarding fasting and detoxification appeared in the *American Journal of Industrial Medicine* in 1984.[20] This study involved patients who had ingested rice oil contaminated with polychlorinated-biphenyls (PCBs). All patients reported improvement in symptoms (primarily involving the nervous system including depression, inability to concentrate, tingling sensations, and fatigue) and some observed dramatic relief, after undergoing 7 to 10 day fasts. This research supports the therapeutic effects of fasting as an aid to detoxification.

Note that caution must be used when fasting. Please consult a physician before going on any unsupervised fast.

If you elect to try a fast, it is a good idea to support your body's detoxification reactions while fasting, especially if, for example, you suffer from impaired liver function (see above) or have a long history of exposure to fat-soluble toxins such as pesticides, cleaning solvents, and formaldehyde. During a fast, stored toxins in our fat cells are released into the system. For example, the pesticide DDT has been shown to be mobilized during a fast and may reach blood levels toxic to the nervous system.[6]

A three-day fresh juice fast can better support detoxification reactions than a water fast or a longer fast. Longer fasts require strict medical supervision while a short fast can usually be conducted at home, rather than at an inpatient facility. Before starting an unsupervised fast, however, remember to consult your physician.

A three-day juice fast consists of three or four 8- to 12-ounce juice meals spread throughout the day. During this period, your body will begin ridding itself of stored toxins. Drinking fresh juice reduces some of the side effects associated with a water fast, such as light-headedness, tiredness, headaches, and so on. While on a fresh juice fast, individuals typically experience an increased sense of well-being, renewed energy, clearer thoughts, and a sense of purity.

To further aid in detoxification, follow these guidelines:

1. Take a high-potency multiple vitamin and mineral formula to provide general support.

2. Take a lipotropic formula according to the guidelines above.

3. Take 1,000 mg of vitamin C three times daily.

4. Take 1 to 2 tablespoons of a fiber supplement at night before retiring. The best fiber sources are the water-soluble fibers such as powdered psyllium seed husks, guar gum, oat bran, and so on.

5. If your body is particularly high in toxins, take silymarin at a dosage of 70 to 210 mg three times daily.

Other Tips on Fasting   Although a short juice fast can be started at any time, it is best to begin on a weekend or during a time period when adequate rest can be assured. The more rest, the better the results because energy can be directed toward healing instead of other bodily functions.

Prepare for a fast by making your last solid meal (the day before the fast) one of only fresh fruits and vegetables (some authorities recommend a full day of raw food to start a fast, even a juice fast).

Only fresh fruit and vegetable juices (ideally prepared from organic produce) should be consumed for the next three to five days. Four 8- to 12-ounce glasses of fresh juice should be consumed throughout the day. In addition to the fresh juice, pure water should also be consumed. The quantity of water consumed should be dictated by thirst, but at least four 8-ounce glasses should be consumed every day during the fast.

Do not drink coffee, bottled, canned, or frozen juice, or soft drinks. Herbal teas can be quite supportive during a fast, but they should not be sweetened.

Exercise is not usually encouraged while fasting. It is a good idea to conserve your energy to allow maximum healing. Short walks or light stretching can be useful, but heavy workouts tax the system and inhibit repair and elimination.

Rest is one of the most important aspects of a fast. A nap or two during the day is recommended. Less sleep will usually be required at night, since your daily activity is less than normal. Body temperature usually drops during a fast, as does blood pressure and pulse and respiratory rate—all measures of the slowing of the metabolic rate of the body. It is important, therefore, to stay warm.

When it is time to break your fast, it is important to reintroduce solid foods gradually by limiting portions. Do not overeat. Eat slowly, chew thoroughly, and eat foods at room temperature.

Supporting Detoxification by Promoting Elimination

In addition to supporting liver function, proper detoxification also involves promoting proper elimination. The dietary recommendations given in Chapter 4 should be sufficient to promote proper elimination by supplying an ample amount of dietary fiber. If additional support is needed, consider using fiber formulas that act as bulking agents. These formulas can be composed of natural plant fibers derived from psyllium seed, kelp, agar, pectin, and plant gums such as karaya and guar. Or they can be purified semi-synthetic polysaccharides such as methylcellulose and carboxymethyl cellulose sodium.

Psyllium-containing laxatives are the most popular and usually the most effective. Fiber formulas are the laxatives that most closely approximate the natural mechanism which promotes a bowel movement. In the treatment of candidiasis, I generally recommend 3 to 5 grams of soluble fiber at bedtime—especially if anti-yeast therapies are employed—to ensure that dead yeast cells are excreted and not absorbed.

Final Comments

In cases of chronic candidiasis where fatigue and multiple chemical sensitivities are a problem, I often recommend performing a liver detoxification profile in order to diagnose more accurately the disruption of the liver's normal detoxification pathways. A liver detoxification profile is a laboratory test designed to assess the liver's ability to detoxify different chemicals. The test involves analyzing saliva samples following the ingestion of a premeasured amount of caffeine and urine samples after the ingestion of acetaminophen (Tylenol), benzoic acid, and/or aspirin. The liver's ability to detoxify these compounds will be apparent based on the metabolites produced in the saliva and urine.

Laboratories that provide this often necessary battery of tests are Great Smokies Diagnostic Laboratory (1-800-522-4762), National BioTech Laboratory (1-800-846-6285), Diagnos-Techs (1-800-87-TESTS), and Meridian Valley Clinical Laboratory (1-206-859-8700). All of these laboratories provide general guidelines for addressing the abnormalities noted.

8

Probiotics

Probiotics (meaning "for life") is a term used to signify the health-promoting effects of friendly bacteria. There are at least 400 different species of microflora living in the human gastrointestinal tract. The most important friendly bacteria are *Lactobacillus acidophilus* and *Bifidobacterium bifidum* because of the beneficial effects they exert on enhancing immune function and against cancer. Therefore, this chapter shall focus on the principle uses of commercial probiotic supplements containing either *L. acidophilus* or *B. bifidum* or both, as well as fructo-oligosaccharides—a special type of sugar molecule that promotes the growth of health-promoting bacteria.

Historical Perspective

Foods fermented with lactobacilli have been, and still are, of great importance to the diets of most of the world's people. Most cultures use some form of fermented food in their diet such as yogurt, cheese, miso, and tempeh. The symbiotic relationship between humankind and lactobacilli has a long history of important nutritional and therapeutic benefits.

At the turn of the century, the noted Russian scientist Elie Metchnikoff believed that yogurt was the elixir of life.[1] His theory was that putrefactive bacteria in the large intestine produce toxins which invite disease and shorten life. He believed that eating yogurt would cause the lactobacilli to become dominant in the colon and displace the putrefactive bacteria. For years, these claims of healthful effects from fermented foods were considered unscientific folklore. However, a substantial and growing body of scientific evidence has demonstrated that lactobacilli and fermented foods do play a significant role in maintaining human health.

People are not born with lactobacilli in their gastrointestinal tract. Colonization of gram-positive lactobacilli begins after birth, whereupon there is a dramatic increase in their concentration. *B. bifidum* is first introduced through breast feeding to the sterile gut of the infant, and large numbers are soon observed in the feces. Later, other bacteria (including such beneficial strains as *L. casei, L. fermentum, L. salivores, L. brevis,* and so on) become established in the gut through contact with the world. Unfortunately, other, potentially toxic, bacteria also eventually cultivate the colon.[2]

Available Forms of Probiotics

In order to provide benefit, products containing *L. acidophilus* and *B. bifidum* must provide live organisms in such a manner that they survive the hostile environment of the gastrointestinal tract. Several factors—such as species,

Table 8.1 Lactobacilli Found in the Human Intestine

L. acidophilus	L. fermentum
L. bifidus (Bifidobacterium bifidum)	L. leichmannii
L. brevis	L. plantarum
L. casei	L. salivores
L. cellobiosus	

strain, adherence, growth media, and diet—are involved in successful colonization.[3,4]

Typically, a high-quality commercial probiotic preparation will produce greater colonization than simply eating yogurt. One of the key reasons is that yogurt is usually made with *L. bulgaricus* or *Streptococcus thermophilus*. While these two bacteria are friendly and possess some health benefits, they are only transient visitors to the gastrointestinal tract and do not colonize the colon.

Proper manufacturing, packaging, and storing of the probiotic product is necessary to ensure viability, the right amount of moisture, and freedom from contamination. Lactobacilli do not respond well to freeze-drying (lyophilization), spray drying, or conventional frozen storage. Excessive temperatures during packaging or storage can dramatically reduce viability. Also, unless the product has been shown to be stable, refrigeration is necessary. Some products do not have to be refrigerated until after the bottle has been opened.

While a number of excellent companies are providing high-quality probiotic products, it is difficult to sort through all the manufacturers' claims of superiority; indeed, some products have been shown to contain no active *L. acidophilus* at all. A study conducted at the University of Washington concluded, "Most of the lactobacilli-containing products currently available [1990] either do not contain the Lactobacillus species advertised and/or contain other bacteria of questionable benefit."[5]

I feel most confident recommending products that have been developed by Professor Khem M. Shahani, Ph.D., of the University of Nebraska. Dr. Shahani is considered the world's foremost expert on probiotics and is the developer of the DDS-1 strain of *L. acidophilus*—often referred to as the "super-strain" because it exerts benefits far greater than that of the other more than 200 strains of *L. acidophilus.* The author of over 190 scientific studies on the role of lactobacilli in human health, Dr. Shahani has personally endorsed several products available in health food stores.

Principle Uses of Probiotics

The intestinal flora plays a major role in the health of the host.[2-4,6] The intestinal flora is intimately involved in the host's nutritional status and affects immune-system function, cholesterol metabolism, carcinogenesis, and aging. Due to the importance of *L. acidophilus* and *B. bifidum* to human health, probiotic supplements of these bacteria can be used to promote overall good health. There are several specific uses for probiotics. The four primary areas of use related to the treatment of chronic candidiasis are promoting a healthy intestinal environment, using probiotics as post-antibiotic therapy, treating vaginal yeast infections, and resolving urinary tract infections.

Promoting a Healthy Intestinal Environment

Lactobacilli have long been noted for the role they play in the prevention of and defense against diseases, particularly those of the gastrointestinal tract and vagina. As part of the normal flora of the body, they inhibit the growth of other organisms in a number of ways: through competition for nutrients, alteration of pH and oxygen tension to levels less favorable to pathogens (disease-causing organisms), prevention of attachment of pathogens by physically covering attachment sites, and production of limiting factors such as anti-microbial factors.[2-4,6]

Lactobacilli produce a variety of limiting factors that inhibit or antagonize other bacteria. These include metabolic end products such as organic acids (lactic and acetic acid), hydrogen peroxide, and compounds known as bacteriocins.[7-18] Although some researchers have isolated substances from lactobacilli which they have labeled antibiotics, these are probably more accurately described as *bacteriocins.* Bacteriocins are proteins that are produced by certain bacteria which exert a lethal effect on closely related bacteria. In general, bacteriocins have a narrower range of activity than antibiotics, but are often more lethal.

Some of the anti-microbial activity of *L. acidophilus* has been shown to be due to its production of hydrogen peroxide.[17,18] (This reaction requires an ample supply of folic acid and riboflavin.) In addition to these direct effects, some researchers believe that the anti-microbial activity of *L. acidophilus* is also due to immune-system stimulation.[19-24]

The earliest reported therapeutic uses of *L. acidophilus*, in the 1920s, suggested that their proliferation was associated with a concomitant decrease in potentially harmful coliform bacteria. This effect has since been confirmed.[25-27] However, it is believed that many of the earlier commercial products were less reliable than those used in later published clinical trials because of inappropriate strains and problems with production, storage, and distribution to consumers.[28]

Table 8.2   Bacteria and Yeast Inhibited by *L. acidophilus*

Bacillus subtillis	*Proteus vulgaris*
B. cerus	*Pseudomonas aeruginosa*
B. stearothermophilus	*P. flourescens*
Candida albicans	*Salmonella typhosa*
Clostridium perfringens	*S. schottmuelleri*
E. coli	*Shigella dysenteriae*
Klebsiella pneumoniae	*S. paradysenteriae*
L. bulgaricus	*Sarcina lutea*
L. fermentum	*Serratia marcescens*
L. helveticus	*Staphylococcus aureus*
L. lactis	*Streptococcus fecalis*
L. leichmannii	*S. lactis*
L. plantarium	*Vibrio comma*

Post-Antibiotic Therapy

Acidophilus supplementation is particularly important for preventing and treating antibiotic-induced diarrhea. *L. acidophilus* has been shown to correct the increase of potentially harmful bacteria (e.g., an overgrowth of gram-negative bacteria) observed following the administration of broad-spectrum antibiotics or as occurs with any acute or chronic diarrhea.[2-4,29-31] Similarly, a mixture of *Bifidobacterium bifidum* and *L. acidophilus* inhibited the lowering of fecal flora induced by ampicillin and maintained the equilibrium of the intestinal ecosystem.[29]

Although it is commonly believed that acidophilus supplements are not effective if taken during antibiotic therapy, research actually supports the use of *L. acidophilus* during antibiotic administration.[29,30] Reduction of friendly bacteria and/or superinfection with antibiotic-resistant flora may be prevented by administering *L. acidophilus* products during antibiotic therapy. A dosage of at least 15 to 20 billion organisms is required. I would still recommend taking the probiotic supplement as far away from the antibiotic as possible. For example if the antibiotic is to be taken three times daily with meals, I would recommend the probiotic be taken between meals or at night before retiring.

Treating Yeast Infections

L. acidophilus has been shown to retard the growth of *Candida albicans*—the major yeast involved in vaginal yeast infections.[32] *L. acidophilus* is a normal constituent of the vaginal flora, where it contributes to the maintenance of the acid pH by fermenting vaginal glycogen to lactic acid.[33-36]

Suppression of *L. acidophilus* by broad-spectrum antibiotics leads to the overgrowth of yeast and other bacteria.[37] Clinical studies have suggested that the introduction of yogurt or lactobacilli to the vagina can assist in clearing up and preventing recurrent vaginal yeast infections as well as bacterial vaginosis.[38] (For more information on the use of *L. acidophilus* in treating vaginal yeast infections, see Chapter 10, page 133).

Resolving Urinary Tract Infections

One of the problems with antibiotic therapy for urinary tract infections (i.e., bladder infections) is that it disturbs the bacterial flora that protect against urinary tract infections, thus leading to recurrent infections. The insertion of lactobacilli suppositories into the vagina after treatment with antibiotics has been shown to significantly reduce the recurrence rate of bladder infections.[39] Women given antibiotics should routinely reestablish proper vaginal flora by following the guidelines given in Chapter 10, page 133. Oral therapy with lactobacilli supplements at the dosages given on page 120 is also a good idea.

Fructo-Oligosaccharides

Food components that may help to promote the growth of friendly bacteria include fructo-oligosaccharides (FOS). These short-chain polysaccharides are just now entering the U.S. market but they are extremely popular overseas. For example, the Japanese market for FOS exceeded $46 million in 1990 and the number of Japanese consumer products containing purified FOS reached 450 in 1991.[40]

FOS is not digested by humans. Instead it feeds the friendly bacteria. Human studies have shown that FOS increases bifidobacteria and lactobacilli while simultaneously reducing the colonies of detrimental bacteria. Other benefits noted with FOS supplementation include increased production of beneficial short-chain fatty acids, such as butyrate; improved liver function; reduction of serum cholesterol and blood pressure; and improved elimination of toxic compounds.[40,41]

The dosage recommendation for pure FOS is 2,000 to 3,000 mg daily for a period of one month or as long as desired. Natural food sources of FOS include Jerusalem artichokes, onions, asparagus, and garlic. However, the estimated average daily ingestion of FOS from food sources is estimated to be 800 mg. Thus, supplementation with FOS may be necessary to help boost FOS intake and promote the growth of friendly bacteria—especially bifidobacteria.[41]

Final Comments

The appropriate dosage of a commercial probiotic supplement is based upon the number of live organisms that it contains. The ingestion of 1 to 10 billion viable *L. aci-*

dophilus or *B. bifidum* cells daily is a sufficient dosage for most people. Amounts exceeding this may induce mild gastrointestinal disturbances, while smaller amounts may not be able to colonize the gastrointestinal tract. Therapy should be at least one month in length, but can be continued indefinitely if so desired.

9

Natural and Prescription
Anti-Yeast Agents

This chapter will discuss several natural and prescription anti-yeast agents. In my experience most patients (although not all) can achieve benefits from the natural agents described here rather than using the drug approach. Use of any anti-yeast therapy without the supplemental support discussed below will likely result in the *Herxheimer reaction* due to the rapid killing of the candida organism and the body's subsequent absorption of large quantities of yeast toxins, cell particles, and antigens. The Herxheimer reaction refers to a worsening of symptoms as a result of this die-off of candida. The Herxheimer reaction can be minimized by:

1. Following the dietary recommendations given in Chapter 4 for a minimum of two weeks before taking an anti-yeast agent.
2. Supporting your liver by following the recommendations given in Chapter 7.

3. Starting any of the anti-yeast medications described below in low dosages and gradually increasing the dosages over one month to the full therapeutic dosage.

Natural Anti-Yeast Agents

A number of natural agents have proven activity against *Candida albicans.* Rather than relying on these agents as a primary therapy, however, it is important to address the factors that predispose one to chronic candidiasis, especially lack of either hydrochloric acid or pancreatic enzymes (these were discussed in Chapter 3).

The four approaches that I feel most comfortable in recommending as natural agents against *Candida albicans* are:

Caprylic acid

Berberine-containing plants

Garlic

Enteric-coated volatile oil preparations

Caprylic Acid

Caprylic acid, a naturally occurring fatty acid, has been reported to be an effective anti-fungal compound in the treatment of candidiasis.[1,2] Because caprylic acid is readily absorbed by the intestines, it is necessary to take time-released or enteric-coated formulas in order to allow for gradual release throughout the entire intestinal tract.[3] The standard dosage for these delayed-release preparations is 1,000 to 2,000 mg with meals for a minimum of one month (or until absence of symptoms or the presence of *Candida albicans* is not detected in a stool culture).

Berberine-Containing Plants

Berberine-containing plants include goldenseal (*Hydrastis canadensis*), barberry (*Berberis vulgaris*), Oregon grape (*Berberis aquifolium*), and goldthread (*Coptis chinensis*). Berberine, an alkaloid, has been extensively studied in both experimental and clinical settings for its antibiotic activity. Berberine exhibits a broad spectrum of antibiotic activity against bacteria, protozoa, and fungi, including *Candida albicans.*[4–10]

Berberine's antibiotic action against some pathogens (disease-producing organisms) is actually stronger than that of antibiotics that are commonly used to treat the diseases that these pathogens cause. Berberine's action in inhibiting *Candida albicans,* as well as pathogenic bacteria, prevents the overgrowth of yeast that is a common side effect of antibiotic use.

Diarrhea is a common symptom in patients with chronic candidiasis. Berberine has shown remarkable anti-diarrheal activity in even the most severe cases. Positive clinical results have been shown with berberine in relieving diarrhea in cases of cholera, amebiasis, giardiasis, and other causes of acute gastrointestinal infection (e.g., *E. coli,* shigella, salmonella, and klebsiella) and may also relieve the diarrhea seen in patients with chronic candidiasis.[11–19]

The dosage of any berberine-containing plant should be based on berberine content. Because there is a wide range of quality in berberine-containing plant preparations, standardized extracts are preferred. Take the following dosages three times a day for a minimum of one month (or until the absence of symptoms or the presence of *Candida albicans* is not detected in a stool culture):

Dried root or as infusion (tea): 2 to 4 grams

Tincture (1:5): 6 to 12 ml (1½ to 3 tsp)

Fluid extract (1:1): 2 to 4 ml (½ to 1 tsp)

Solid (powdered dry) extract (4:1 or 8% to 12% alkaloid content): 250 to 500 mg

The above dosages will result in consumption of 25 to 50 mg of berberine three times daily or a daily dosage of up to 150 mg. For children a dosage based on body weight is appropriate. That is, the daily dosage should be the equivalent to 5 to 10 mg of berberine per kg (2.2 pounds) of body weight.

Berberine and berberine-containing plants are generally nontoxic at the recommended dosages, however, berberine-containing plants are *not* recommended for use during pregnancy and higher dosages may interfere with B-vitamin metabolism.[20]

Garlic

Garlic has demonstrated significant anti-fungal activity. In fact, its inhibition of *Candida albicans* has been shown to be more potent than nystatin, gentian violet, and six other reputed anti-fungal agents.[21-23] The active component in garlic is allicin.

Modern clinical use of garlic features the use of commercial preparations designed to offer the benefits of garlic without the odor. These are prepared in such a manner that the allicin (which is a pungent and odorous compound) is not formed until the enteric-coated tablet is delivered to the small and large intestines.

In the treatment of chronic candidiasis, I generally recommend a daily dosage of at least 10 mg of allicin or a total allicin potential of 4,000 mcg. This amount is equal to approximately 1 clove (4 grams) of fresh, raw garlic. Going beyond this dosage with the commercial preparations usually results in a detectable odor of garlic. Like other natural anti-candida therapies, treatment should be continued for a minimum of one month (or until absence of symptoms or the presence of *Candida albicans* is not detected in a stool culture).

Enteric-Coated Volatile Oils

The most recent natural anti-candida formulas are enteric-coated volatile-oil preparations. Volatile oils from oregano, thyme, peppermint, and rosemary are very powerful anti-fungal agents. A recent study compared the anti-candida effect of oregano oil to caprylic acid.[24] The results indicated that the anti-candida activity of oregano oil was over 100 times more potent than caprylic acid. Because volatile oils are quickly absorbed, as well as associated with inducing heartburn, an enteric coating is recommended to ensure delivery to the small and large intestine.

An effective dosage for an enteric-coated volatile-oil preparation is 0.2 to 0.4 ml twice daily between meals for a minimum of one month (or until absence of symptoms or presence of *Candida albicans* is not detected in a stool culture).

Prescription Anti-Yeast Therapies

The two primary categories of prescription anti-yeast therapies are nystatin and the azole drugs. Often these drugs are combined to compensate for their individual weaknesses.

Nystatin

Nystatin is a naturally occurring anti-fungal agent derived from another yeast (*Streptomyces noursei*) that grows in the soil. Nystatin has become the most widely used prescription anti-candida medication. It is an extremely safe drug primarily because it is so poorly absorbed. This poor absorption limits its effectiveness in many cases because it appears to be unable to eradicate candida organisms that have become firmly entrenched in the lining of the gastrointestinal tract. Nonetheless, nystatin is effective in reducing many of the symptoms of chronic candidiasis—particularly those that involve the gastrointestinal tract.

The Azole Drugs

The azole drugs—including ketoconazole (Nizoral), fluconazole (Diflucan), and itraconazole (Sporanox)—have become quite popular in the treatment of candida infections in conventional as well as in alternative medical circles. All three of these drugs are completely absorbed by the gastrointestinal tract and are associated with liver damage (which occurs in roughly 1 in 100 individuals). Although rare, severe liver damage (1 in 10,000) and even death has resulted from the use of these drugs.

Unfortunately, there appears to be no way of determining who is likely to suffer such serious consequences. In cases of serious liver damage, researchers have not found any obvious relationship between total daily dose, duration of therapy, age, sex, or any other associative factor. Despite the potential problems these drugs can cause, they are powerful anti-candida agents. It seems that some patients will respond to them and no other measures. However, because of the risks, I recommend reserving their use as a "last-ditch" effort for patients with severe chronic candidiasis. When these drugs are used, it is important to check liver enzymes in the blood to determine if any liver damage is occurring.

Diflucan and Sporanox seem to be safer choices than Nizoral. Diflucan appears to be slightly more effective than Sporanox in treating chronic intestinal candidiasis, but Sporanox is more effective than Diflucan if there is also skin or nail involvement. Many physicians prescribe a combination of an azole anti-fungal and nystatin. The primary reason is that since the azole drugs are so well-absorbed and reabsorbed by the intestines, it is often difficult to achieve sufficient concentrations in the colon to effectively eradicate candida from this tissue. Nystatin appears to compensate for this shortcoming.

Final Comments

As I've discussed throughout this book, a comprehensive approach is more effective in treating chronic candidiasis than simply trying to kill the candida with a drug. Drugs such as nystatin and the azole drugs rarely produce significant long-term results on their own because they fail to address the underlying factors which promoted the candida overgrowth in the first place. It is like trying to weed your garden by simply cutting the weeds instead of pulling them out by the roots.

Nonetheless, in many cases it is useful to try to eradicate *Candida albicans* from your system with the help of these drugs. My latest approach in these cases is to use an enteric-coated volatile oil preparation (such as Candida Formula from Enzymatic Therapy or, previous to this product's introduction, Peppermint Plus from Enzymatic Therapy or ADP from Biotics Research Laboratories) along with an enteric-coated fresh garlic preparation (such as Garlinase 4000). I have found this approach to be effective in most cases.

In more difficult cases, I recommend using the enteric-coated volatile oil preparation and garlic in combination with the prescription drug nystatin (because this drug is naturally derived, naturopathic physicians in my state can legally prescribe it). A follow-up stool culture and candida-antigen determination will confirm if the candida has been eliminated. If it has and symptoms are still apparent, it is likely that they are unrelated to an overgrowth of *Candida albicans.* Similar symptoms can be caused by small intestinal bacterial overgrowth. In this scenario, I tend to use pancreatic enzymes and berber-ine-containing plants such as goldenseal in an attempt to resolve the problem.

10

Special Concerns for Women: Vaginal Yeast Infections, Vulvodynia, and Premenstrual Syndrome

Chronic candidiasis affects women roughly four times more often than men. The primary reasons are that (1) women use antibiotics more extensively as a result of urinary tract infections and acne; (2) many women are on birth control pills, which can disrupt the normal vaginal environment; (3) hormonal changes during the menstrual cycle can alter the pH of the vagina; and (4) the vaginal tract can be a very hospitable environment for *Candida albicans*. Because yeast overgrowth is often an underlying factor in many female complaints, this chapter will look at the role of chronic candidiasis in vaginal yeast infections, vulvodynia, and premenstrual syndrome.

Vaginal Yeast Infections

The relative frequency and the total incidence of vaginal yeast infections (candidal vaginitis) has increased dramatically in the past 40 years. Several factors have contributed to this increased incidence (see Table 10.1), chief among them being the increased use of antibiotics. The problem of vaginal yeast infections resulting from antibiotic use are well-known by virtually every woman. The alterations that antibiotics cause in both intestinal and vaginal flora favor the growth of candida. Steroids, oral contraceptives, and the continuing increase in diabetes mellitus also have contributed to the growing problem of vaginal yeast infections.

In general, it can be stated that vaginal yeast infections arise from a disturbance to the ecology of the healthy vagina. Factors influencing the vaginal environment include the pH, glycogen content, glucose level, the presence of other organisms (particularly lactobacilli), the natural flushing action of vaginal secretions, the presence of blood, and the presence of antibodies and other compounds in the vaginal secretions.

Immune dysfunction will predispose a woman to increased vaginal yeast infections. Depressed immunity may occur as a result of nutritional deficiencies, medications (e.g., steroids), pregnancy, or serious illness. Other factors may predispose one to vaginal yeast infections: diabetes mellitus, the wearing of synthetic pantyhose (which tend to retain moisture), and pregnancy. Yeast infections are three times more prevalent in women wearing pantyhose than those wearing cotton underwear, because the pantyhose prevent drying of the area.[1]

Table 10.1   Predisposing Factors to Candidal Vaginitis

Allergies	Oral contraceptives
Antibiotics	Pantyhose
Diabetes mellitus	Pregnancy
Elevated vaginal pH	Steroids
Gastrointestinal candidiasis	

Most cases of recurrent candidal vaginitis are due either to transmission of candida from the gastrointestinal tract or failure to recognize and treat the presence of one or more predisposing factors. In extremely persistent cases, sexual partners may be a source of reinfection. Allergies have also been reported to cause recurrent candidiasis, which resolves when the allergies are treated.[2]

Signs and Symptoms of Vaginal Yeast Infections

The primary symptom of a vaginal yeast infection is vulvar itching, which can be quite severe. This is associated with the presence of a thick, curdy ("cottage-cheesy") discharge, which may reveal pinpoint bleeding when removed. The presence of such a discharge is strong evidence of a yeast infection, but its absence does not rule out candida.

Treating Vaginal Yeast Infections

Successfully treating vaginal yeast infections involves reestablishing the normal vaginal flora. In particular, it is very important to reestablish the adequate presence of *Lactobacillus acidophilus*. These desirable bacteria are an integral component of the normal vaginal flora and help to maintain a healthy vaginal ecology by preventing the overgrowth of *Candida albicans* and less desirable bacterial species. As thoroughly discussed in Chapter 8, *L. acidophilus* does this by producing lactic acid and natural antibiotic substances. In addition, *L. acidophilus* competes with other bacteria and *Candida albicans* for the utilization of glucose.

Lactobacilli Reestablishment of normal vaginal lactobacilli can be accomplished by douching twice a day with a solution containing acidophilus. The solution is best prepared by using a high-quality acidophilus supplement or

active-culture yogurt (careful reading of labels is important, since most commercially available yogurts do not
use lactobacilli). Dissolve enough of either choice in 10 ml
(roughly 2 tablespoons) of water to provide 1 billion
organisms. Use a syringe to douche the material into the
vagina. Since lactobacilli are normal inhabitants of the
vaginal flora, the douche can be retained in the vagina as
long as desired. Douching twice weekly for four weeks
should be enough to reestablish normal vaginal flora.

In addition, I recommend taking an oral probiotic supplement according to the guidelines presented in Chapter
8. Also, remember that whenever antibiotics (particularly
broad-spectrum ones) are taken for any reason, regular
use of a probiotic supplement and anti-yeast agents will
reduce the risk of complications, such as diarrhea and
candida overgrowth.

Iodine Iodine used topically as a douche is effective
against a wide range of infectious agents linked to vaginal
infections, including *Candida albicans.* Povidone iodine
(Betadine) has all the advantages of iodine without the
disadvantages of stinging and staining. Betadine is available over the counter at any pharmacy. A study published
in 1969 found that povidone iodine was effective in treating 100% of cases of candidal vaginitis, 80% of tricho-
monas, and 93% of combination infections. A douching
solution diluted to 1 part iodine in 100 parts water used
twice daily for 14 days is effective against most organisms.[3-7] However, excessive use must be avoided because
some iodine will be absorbed into the system and can
cause suppression of thyroid function.

Boric Acid Capsules of boric acid inserted into the vagina
have been used to treat candidiasis with success rates
equal to or better than those of nystatin and creams
containing miconazole, clotrimazole, or butoconazole.[8-10]

Table 10.2 Outcome of Therapy with Conventional Anti-fungal Agents Versus Boric Acid

Agent	Loss of symptoms (% of patients)	Abnormal microscopic findings (% of patients)
Anti-fungals	52	100
Boric acid	98	2

Data from Meeker, C. I.: "Candidiasis: An Obstinate Problem." *Med Times* 106:26–32, 1978.

Boric-acid treatment offers an inexpensive, easily accessible therapy for vaginal yeast infections. In a recent study of 92 women with chronic vaginal yeast infections (see Table 10.2), boric-acid treatment was shown to be significantly more effective in relieving symptoms and killing yeast than prescription anti-fungal drugs.[10] In fact, no patient receiving anti-fungal drugs had a normal microscopic exam. All exams in these patients demonstrated continued presence of yeast, damaged cells that line the vagina, or some other abnormality.

The effective dosage was 600 mg of boric acid in a vaginal suppository twice daily for two weeks.

In chronic cases of vaginal yeast infections, standard anti-fungal agents are often ineffective. In these cases, it is recommended that boric acid (600 mg) be used twice a day for four months. After this time further use may not be necessary, but I would recommend continuing to use boric acid during menstruation because the vaginal environment during menses tends to favor an overgrowth of *Candida albicans*.

Side effects with boric acid are quite rare. The most common side effect is burning of the labia due to boric acid leaking out of the vagina. If this occurs, reduce the amount of boric acid or discontinue use.

Gentian Violet   Gentian violet is a dark-purple dye that can kill *Candida albicans.* In fact, it has been stated that swabbing the vagina with gentian violet is "as close to a specific treatment for candida as exists."[10] Despite this proclamation, I prefer other measures because it is extremely messy. If you elect to give it a try, be careful. The best way to apply gentian violet is to soak a tampon in it and then insert the tampon into the vagina. Leave in the vagina for 2 to 3 hours. An application once a day is ample; continue this treatment for 7 to 10 days.

Vulvodynia

The vulva is the external, visible part of the female genitalia. Women with chronic candidiasis may experience itchiness or discomfort, which is referred to as *pruritis vulvae. Vulvodynia,* on the other hand, is described as chronic vulvar discomfort characterized by sensations of burning, stinging, irritation, or rawness. Vulvodynia is different than pruritis vulvae; typically in pruritis vulvae there is redness while in vulvodynia physical signs are typically quite subtle or absent altogether. Because of this absence of physical findings, many women with vulvodynia are told it is "all in their head." Adding to this insult is the fact that vulvodynia is often a factor in *dyspareunia*—the medical term for painful intercourse.

Symptoms of vulvodynia can range from very mild to quite severe. Hypersensitivity along the edge of the small labia is common and can make walking quite painful. Some women are so sensitive that they cannot wear underwear because of the pain or burning discomfort caused by the underwear touching their pubic hair. Other women complain of burning pain across the pubic line, shooting pain through the buttocks or thighs, and stabbing pains into the vagina.

Although not all cases of vulvodynia are related to the yeast syndrome, I have had several patients experience complete resolution of symptoms upon following a yeast-treatment program such as the one described in this book and summarized in Chapter 11. Dr. William Crook, author of *The Yeast Connection and the Woman,* (Professional Books, 1996) reports similar results. Several of my colleagues who specialize in female health issues also report that chronic candidiasis is almost always a factor in vulvodynia and that successful eradication of the yeast often results in clinical improvement.

In addition to measures designed to address chronic candidiasis, there are other natural measures that appear to be quite helpful in treating vulvodynia. Before I discuss these natural measures, I want to encourage any woman with vulvodynia and all physicians to support:

The Vulvar Pain Foundation
Joanne Yount, Executive Director
P.O. Drawer 177
Graham, NC 27253
910-226-0704
FAX 910-226-8518

This nonprofit organization was established in 1992 in order to provide reliable information on vulvar pain to women suffering from vulvodynia as well as their health-care professionals. The Vulvar Pain Foundation publishes a quarterly newsletter and organizes seminars for its members and physicians. The yearly cost for membership is $40. It is well worth supporting.

I first learned of this organization through a patient. The patient also brought with her a packet of information put together by Clive C. Solomons, Ph.D., a former professor and director of biochemical research at the University of Colorado. In the mid-1980s, Dr. Solomons identified oxalate (oxalic acid) as a possible biochemical cause for vulvodynia.

According to Dr. Solomons and his colleagues, the burning pain of vulvodynia is caused largely as a result of high levels of oxalate being excreted in the urine and coming into contact with the vulva or by the production of oxalate as a result of breakdown of skin components in the vulva.[11] Therapy involves two primary recommendations: (1) a low oxalate diet and (2) supplementation with calcium citrate.

Based on Dr. Solomons's clinical research, which shows a 70% success rate, and testimonials from hundreds of women, Joanne Yount, executive director of the Vulvar Pain Foundation, claims that "the low oxalate diet and citrate treatment, when followed consistently over an extended period of time, and especially when followed in accordance with recommendations based on laboratory analyses, is eventually substantially effective for most, though not all, women who use it."

A Low Oxalate Diet

Dietary sources of oxalate can increase the urinary concentration of oxalate. This relationship has been studied most in relation to kidney-stone formation because most kidney stones are composed of calcium oxalate crystals, but it also appears to be important in the treatment of vulvodynia. Avoid high and medium oxalate foods such as spinach and other greens, celery, beets, eggplant, green peppers, berries of all types, beer, chocolate, peanuts, pecans, and tea.

For many years, detractors of high dosages of vitamin C have cautioned that taking too much vitamin C can lead to increased oxalate formation in the urine and possibly increase the risk of kidney stones. However, this concern has been totally disproved. Healthy volunteers given 10 g of vitamin C (2,000 mg five times daily) only increased their mean urinary oxalate levels from about 50 mg to 90 mg per day.[12] Although hardly a matter of concern for most individuals, in women with vulvodynia, I recommend playing it safe and avoiding dosages greater than 500 mg three times daily.

Calcium Citrate

Citrate is a naturally occurring acid that plays a role in the Krebs cycle—the energy-producing cycle that liberates chemical energy from sugars. Citrate also appears to play a role in reducing urinary oxalate levels. Again, this relationship has been most extensively studied in regard to kidney stones. Citrate reduces the urinary saturation of stone-forming calcium salts by forming complexes with calcium and reducing the level of oxalates. It also retards the nucleation and crystalline growth of the calcium salts. If citrate levels are low, this inhibitory activity is not present and stone formation is likely to occur. Decreased urinary citrate is found in 20% to 60% of patients with kidney stones.[13,14]

Citrate supplementation has been shown to be quite successful in preventing recurrent kidney stones.[13,14] Potassium citrate or sodium citrate have been used in clinical studies. A more advantageous salt of citric acid in the prevention of kidney stones would appear to be magnesium citrate. In the treatment of vulvodynia, however, calcium citrate appears to be more advantageous than these other forms based on the preliminary studies conducted by Dr. Solomons.

Many companies market calcium citrate or calcium-magnesium citrate. In general, 200 mg of elemental calcium in a calcium citrate tablet or capsule will provide 750 mg of citrate. The dosage is based upon the level of calcium because the amount of citrate in the product is rarely listed on the label. The dosage of calcium citrate in the treatment of vulvodynia can be determined by first measuring urinary oxalate levels collected at 10 different times during a 24-hour period. This test is performed at Dr. Solomons's lab (Sci-Con, P.O. Box 61386, Denver, CO 80206, telephone 303-388-7140) at a cost of $350 and includes customized treatment recommendations on the timing and dosage of calcium citrate.

However, I recommend doing some trial and error before investing in this test. My reasoning is that it may not be necessary to even perform this test. It is significantly less expensive to follow the low oxalate diet and citrate supplementation plan for four weeks and see what happens. Perhaps an even better reason is illustrated by the following case history.

A Case History

Kathi was a 32-year-old woman who came to see me for her severe vulvodynia. She reported a sharp stabbing pain that radiated from her vulva into her vagina. It was debilitating at times, making it virtually impossible to carry out daily activities. Like many patients whom I see, Kathi had worked with many other physicians and had even performed the urinary oxalate determination and followed the recommendations from Dr. Solomons. Yet her pain was not significantly lessened. As evident from the chart in Figure 10.1 below, her symptoms appeared to be related to urinary oxalate. But the low oxalate diet and citrate supplementation were not providing any real benefit despite her strict adherence to the plan.

Why didn't Kathi respond to the low oxalate diet and citrate supplementation? Kathi's medical history (frequent antibiotic use for urinary tract infections and frequent vaginal yeast infections) and other symptoms strongly suggested that chronic candidiasis was possibly a factor.

Clive C. Solomons, Ph.D.   ***Sci-Con***

Tel (303) 388-7140   PO Box 61386   Date of Urine

Fax (303) 388-7799   Denver, CO 80206-8386   Collection: 5/12/XX

ID Code: XXXX

Patient Name: XXXX

	Time	OX MG%	Pain
1	10:00 A.M.	20.00	1
2	12:45 P.M.	9.00	2
3	3:23 P.M.	5.00	3
4	5:25 P.M.	16.00	5
5	6:50 P.M.	3.00	5
6	8:36 P.M.	10.00	5
7	10:40 P.M.	3.00	5
8	3:20 A.M.	10.00	1
9	7:00 A.M.	3.00	1
10	9:40 A.M.	16.00	2

Citrate is most effective if administered before the occurrence of high peaks of oxalate concentration. The dosages/times most likely to be effective are:

Rx

__*1*__ tabs   Time __*9 a.m.*__

__*2*__ tabs   Time __*5 p.m.*__

__*2*__ tabs   Time __*10 p.m.*__

_____ tabs   Time _____

Most citrate tabs contain approximately 750 mg.

Take on an empty stomach. Allow 20 min. before eating. Do not take antacids containing aluminum.

Urinary Oxalate Concentration and Subjective Pain Assessment

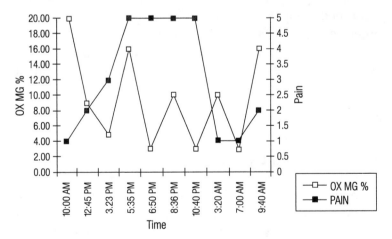

Figure 10.1   Sample Urinary Oxalate Determination

Based upon this, I decided to treat her for candidiasis as well as vulvodynia. The result? Kathi's vulvodynia completely resolved within the first two weeks of treatment. What was her treatment? The dietary plan outlined in Chapter 4 plus the low oxalate diet and the following supplements from Enzymatic Therapy:

> Krebs Cycle Chelates: 1 tablet four times daily
>
> Doctor's Choice for Women: 1 tablet three times daily
>
> Candida Formula: 1 to 2 capsules twice daily between meals
>
> Enzydophilus: 1 capsule three times daily with meals for the first week; thereafter, 1 capsule daily with a meal

Rather than using calcium citrate alone, I used a balanced complete mineral formula where the minerals are bound to the complete Krebs cycle. Other Krebs cycle compounds such as fumarate, malate, succinate, and aspartate produce similar effects to citrate. Specifically, minerals bound to these compounds have been shown to be better absorbed compared to other mineral chelates. Krebs cycle intermediates fulfill every requirement for an optimum mineral chelating agent: (1) they are easily ionized, (2) they are almost completely degraded, (3) they have virtually no toxicity, and (4) they have been shown to increase the absorption of calcium and other minerals.

Premenstrual Syndrome

In addition to vaginal yeast infections and vulvodynia, women with the yeast syndrome tend to suffer more severely from premenstrual syndrome (PMS)—a recurrent condition of women characterized by troublesome symptoms 7 to 14 days before menstruation. Typical symptoms include decreased energy, tension, irritability, depression, headache, altered sex drive, breast pain, backache, abdominal bloating, and edema of the fingers and ankles. PMS is estimated to affect between 30% to 40% of menstruating women with peak occurrences among women in their thirties and forties. In most cases symptoms are relatively mild, however, in about 10% of all women symptoms can be quite severe. Severe PMS with depression, irritability, and severe mood swings is referred to as *premenstrual dysphoric disorder.*

Like the yeast syndrome, PMS represents a multifactorial condition in that no single cause explains PMS in every case. Many factors appear to play a role in PMS, with some factors being more important in one case than another. PMS is thoroughly discussed in my "Getting Well Naturally" series title *Premenstrual Syndrome* (Prima, 1997). If you suffer from PMS, this book provides important direction.

Treating PMS

Here is a brief summary of my key recommendations for treating PMS:

1. Follow a vegetarian or predominantly vegetarian diet.
2. Reduce your intake of fat.
3. Eliminate sugar from your diet.
4. Reduce your exposure to environmental estrogens.
5. Increase your intake of soy foods.
6. Eliminate caffeine from your diet.
7. Keep your salt intake low.

8. Supplement your diet with vitamins and minerals according to the guidelines given in Chapter 5.
9. Select the appropriate herbal support.

Herbal Support

If you have PMS-associated breast pain, infrequent periods, or a history of ovarian cysts take chaste-berry (*Vitex agnus-castus*) extract. The usual dosage of chaste-berry extract (often standardized to contain 0.5% agnuside) in tablet or capsule form is 175 to 225 mg daily. If using the liquid extract, the typical dosage is 2 ml daily.

If you typically experience menstrual cramps, take angelica (also known as *dong quai*). I generally recommend that angelica be taken beginning on day 14 of your cycle and continued until menstruation unless you typically experience dysmenorrhea (painful menstruation) in which case I recommend that it be continued until menstruation has stopped. Take the following dosage three times per day:

Powdered root or as a tea: 1 to 2 g

Tincture (1:5): 4 ml (1 tsp)

Fluid extract: 1 ml (¼ tsp)

If you are bothered by PMS water retention, take licorice root (*Glycyrrhiza glabra*). The dosage recommendations below are to be taken three times per day beginning on day 14 of your cycle and continued until menstruation:

Powdered root: 1 to 2 grams

Fluid extract (1:1): 4 ml (1 tsp)

Solid (dry powdered) extract (4:1): 250 to 500 mg

If you suffer from uterine fibroids, take black cohosh (*Cimicifuga racemosa*). Take one tablet twice daily to provide a daily dose of 2 mg of 27-deoxyacteine.

When to Consult a Physician

If you've carefully followed the above treatment recommendations for at least three complete periods and you are not experiencing a significant improvement or complete resolution of your symptoms, further support is indicated. Consult a physician (referral services given on page 9) familiar with nutritional therapies for PMS. The physician should help in identifying possible causative factors and more effective treatment strategies tailored specifically to your case.

Final Comments

Because chronic candidiasis often involves troublesome yet vague symptoms, women with chronic candidiasis are not taken seriously by many physicians. This is most unfortunate. Chronic candidiasis is a real clinical entity. Physicians who discount its significance or downplay its role as a possible causative factor in the special considerations discussed in this chapter do a great disservice to their patients. Chronic candidiasis definitely plays a role in many cases of chronic vaginal infections, vulvodynia, and PMS. Failure to address the intestinal candida issue makes effective treatment of these conditions unlikely. Conversely, addressing the intestinal candida overgrowth issue effectively in these situations often results in a complete resolution of symptoms.

11

Putting It All Together

In the course of this book, I've discussed the many different factors that can predispose one to the yeast syndrome. Because chronic candidiasis is a multifactorial syndrome, it is essential that all of the causal factors be addressed before successful treatment of this condition can be achieved. Although you may feel slightly overwhelmed at this point, many of the recommendations in this book, such as dietary changes, will soon become second nature, especially once you've experienced a renewed feeling of well-being. Following is a comprehensive step-by-step review of the natural approach to the successful elimination of chronic candidiasis.

Step 1: Identify and Address Predisposing Factors

- Eliminate the use of antibiotics, steroids, immune-suppressing drugs, and birth control pills (unless there is absolute medical necessity).

- Consult a physician to determine if you have decreased digestive secretions or follow the recommendations given in Chapter 3.

Step 2: Follow the Candida Control Diet

- Do not eat refined or simple sugars.
- Do not drink milk or consume other dairy products.
- Do not eat foods with a high content of yeast or mold including alcoholic beverages, cheeses, dried fruits, melons, and peanuts.
- Avoid all known or suspected food allergens.

Step 3: Provide Nutritional Support

- Take a high-potency multiple vitamin and mineral formula.
- Take additional antioxidants.
- Take one tablespoon of flaxseed oil daily.

Step 4: Support Immune Function

- Do your best to be a positive, happy person.
- Deal with stress by using positive rather than negative stress-coping techniques.
- Avoid alcohol, sugar, smoking, and elevated cholesterol levels, which can impair immune function.
- Get plenty of rest and good sleep.
- Support your thymus-gland function by taking 750 mg of crude polypeptide fractions daily.

Step 5: Promote Detoxification and Elimination

- Take 3 to 5 grams of a water-soluble fiber source such as guar gum, psyllium seed, or pectin every night.
- If necessary, take lipotropic factors and silymarin to enhance liver function (see Chapter 7 for guidelines).

Step 6: Take Probiotics

- Ingest 1 to 10 billion viable *L. acidophilus* and *B. bifidum* cells daily.

Step 7: Use Appropriate Anti-Yeast Therapy

- Ideally, use the nutritional and herbal supplements recommended in this book to help control against yeast overgrowth and promote a healthy bacterial flora.
- If necessary, see a physician for a prescription anti-yeast drug.

These seven simple steps should resolve chronic candidiasis in most cases. If you follow the guidelines in this book and fail to achieve significant improvement or complete resolution, I strongly urge you to contact one of the organizations listed in Chapter 1 (page 9) in order to find a physician in your area knowledgeable about chronic candidiasis.

References

Chapter 1: An Overview of Chronic Candidiasis (the Yeast Syndrome)

1. Truss O: The Missing Diagnosis. P.O.B. 26508, Birmingham, AL, 1983.
2. Crook WG: The Yeast Connection, 2nd ed. Professional Books, Jackson, TN, 1984.
3. Kroker GF: Chronic candidiasis and allergy. In: Food Allergy and Intolerance. Brostoff J and Challacombe SJ (eds). WB Saunders, Philadelphia, 1987, pp. 850–72.
4. Crook WG: The Yeast Connection and the Woman. Professional Books, Jackson, TN, 1995.
5. Barrie S: Comprehensive Digestive Stool Analysis. In: A Textbook of Natural Medicine. Pizzorno JE and Murray MT (eds.). Bastyr University Publications, Seattle, WA, 1986.
6. Bauman DS and Hagglund HE: Correlation between certain polysystem chronic complaints and an enzyme immunoassay with antigens of *Candida albicans*. J Advancement Med 4:5–19, 1991.
7. Sawada Y, et al.: Polyamines in the intestinal lumen of patients with small bowel bacterial overgrowth. Biochem Soc Trans 22:392(S), 1994.

8. Henriksson AEK, et al.: Small intestinal bacterial overgrowth in patients with rheumatoid arthritis. Annals Rheumatic Dis 52:503–10, 1993.

9. Bjarnason I, MacPherson A, and Hollander D: Intestinal permeability: An overview. Gastroenterol 108:1566–81, 1995.

10. Bjarnason I: Intestinal permeability. Gut 35:S18–22, 1994.

11. Madara JL, et al.: Structure and function of the intestinal epithelial barrier in health and disease. Monogr Pathol 31:306–24, 1990.

12. Rooney PJ, Jenkins RT, and Buchanan WW: A short review of the relationship between intestinal permeability and inflammatory bowel disease. Clin Exp Rheumatol 8:75–83, 1990.

13. Levine JB and Lukawski-Trubish D: Extraintestinal considerations in inflammatory bowel disease. Gastroenterol Clin North Am 24:633–46, 1995.

Chapter 2: Antibiotics and the Yeast Syndrome

1. Reid G, Bruce AW, and Cook RL: Effect on urogenital flora of antibiotic therapy of urinary tract infection. Scand J Infect Dis 22:43–7, 1990.

2. Lidefelt KJ, Bollgren I, and Nord CE: Changes in periurethral microflora after antimicrobial drugs. Arch Dis Child 66:683–5, 1991.

3. Prodromos PN, Brusch CA, and Ceresia GC: Cranberry juice in the treatment of urinary tract infections. Southwest Med 47:17, 1968.

4. Sternlieb P: Cranberry juice in renal disease. New Engl J Med 268:57, 1963.

5. Moen DV: Observations on the effectiveness of cranberry juice in urinary infections. Wisconsin Med J 61:282, 1962.

6. Kahn DH, et al.: Effect of cranberry juice on urine. J Am Diet Assoc 51:251, 1967.

7. Bodel PT, Cotran R, and Kass EH: Cranberry juice and the antibacterial action of hippuric acid. J Lab Clin Med 54:881, 1959.

8. Sobota AE: Inhibition of bacterial adherence by cranberry juice: Potential use for the treatment of urinary tract infections. J Urology 131:1013–6, 1984.

9. Ofek I, et al.: Anti-escherichia activity of cranberry and blueberry juices. N Engl J Med 324:1599, 1991.

10. Munday PE and Savage S: Cymalon in the management of urinary tract symptoms. Genitourin Med 66:461, 1990.

11. Spooner JB: Alkalinization in the management of cystitis. J Int Med Res 12:30–4, 1984.

12. Merck Index, 10th ed. Merck & Co., Rahway, NJ, 1983. pp112–3, 699.

13. Frohne V: Untersuchungen zur frage der harndesifizierenden wirkungen von barentraubenblatt-extracten. Planta Medica 18:1–25, 1970.

14. Leung A: Encyclopedia of Common Natural Ingredients Used in Food, Drugs, and Cosmetics. John Wiley, New York, 1980.

15. Amin AH, Subbaiah TV, and Abbasi KM: Berberine sulfate: Antimicrobial activity, bioassay, and mode of action. Can J Microbiol 15:1067–76, 1969.

16. Marshall FF and Middleton AW: Eosinophilic cystitis. J Urol 112:225–8, 1974.

17. Goldstein M: Eosinophic cystitis. J Urol 106:854–7, 1972.

18. Palacios AS, Juana AD, Sagarra JM, and Duque RA: Eosinophilic food-induced cystitis. Allergol Et Immunopathol 12:463–9, 1984.

19. Orr PH, et al.: Randomized placebo-controlled trials of antibiotics for acute bronchitis: A critical review of the literature. J Fam Practice 36:507–12, 1993.

20. Gonzales R and Sande M: What will it take to stop physicians from prescribing antibiotics in acute bronchitis? Lancet 345:665, 1995.

21. Rimoldi R, Ginesu F, and Giura R: The use of bromelain in pneumological therapy. Drugs Exp Clin Res 4:55–66, 1978.

22. Ryan R: A double-blind clinical evaluation of bromelains in the treatment of acute sinusitis. Headache 7:13–7, 1967.

23. Michaelsson G, Vahlquist A, and Juhlin L: Serum zinc and retinol-binding protein in acne. Br J Dermatol 96:283–6, 1977.

24. Michaelson G, Juhlin L, and Ljunghall K: A double-blind study of the effect of zinc and oxytetracycline in acne vulgaris. Br J Dermatol 97:561–5, 1977.

25. Cunliffe WJ, et al.: A double-blind trial of a zinc sulphate/citrate complex and tetracycline in the treatment of acne. Br J Dermatol 101:321–5, 1979.

26. Dreno B, et al.: Low doses of zinc gluconate for inflammatory acne. Acta Derm Venereol 69:541–3, 1989.
27. Weimar V, Puhl S, Smith W, and Broeke J: Zinc sulphate in acne vulgaris. Arch Dermatol 114:1776–8, 1978.
28. Woodhead M: Antibiotic resistance. Brit J Hosp Med 56:314–5, 1996.
29. Cohen M: Epidemiology of drug resistance: Implications for a post antibiotic era. Science 257:1050–5, 1992.
30. World Health Organization: Fighting Disease, Fostering Development. Report of the Director General. HMSO, London, 1996.
31. Demling L: Is Crohn's disease caused by antibiotics? Hepato-Gastroenterol 41:549–51, 1994.

Chapter 3: Enhancing Digestive Secretions

1. Boero M, et al.: Candida overgrowth in gastric juice of peptic ulcer subjects on short- and long-term treatment with H_2-receptor antagonists. Digestion 28:158–63, 1983.
2. Barrie SA: Heidelberg pH capsule gastric analysis. In: Pizzorno JE and Murray MT: A Textbook of Natural Medicine. Bastyr University Publications, Seattle, WA, 1985.
3. Bray GW: The hypochlorhydria of asthma in childhood. Br Med. J i:181–97, 1930.
4. Rabinowitch IM: Achlorhydria and its clinical significance in diabetes mellitus. Am J Dig Dis 18:322–33, 1949.
5. Carper WM, et al.: Gallstones, gastric secretion and flatulent dyspepsia. Lancet i:413–5, 1967.
6. Rawls WB and Ancona VC: Chronic urticaria associated with hypochlorhydria or achlorhydria. Rev Gastroent Oct:267–71, 1950.
7. Gianella RA, Broitman SA, and Zamcheck N: Influence of gastric acidity on bacterial and parasitic enteric infections. Ann Int Med 78:271–6, 1973.
8. De Witte TJ, Geerdink PJ, and Lamers CB: Hypochlorhydria and hypergastrinaemia in rheumatoid arthritis. Ann Rheum Dis 38:14–17, 1979.
9. Ryle JA and Barber HW. Gastric analysis in acne rosacea. Lancet ii:1195–6, 1920.

10. Ayres S: Gastric secretion in psoriasis, eczema and dermatitis herpetiformis. Arch Derm Jul:854–9, 1929.

11. Dotevall G and Walan A: Gastric secretion of acid and intrinsic factor in patients with hyper and hypothyroidism. Acta Med Scand 186:529–33, 1969.

12. Howitz J and Schwartz M: Vitiligo, achlorhydria, and pernicious anemia. Lancet i:1331–4, 1971.

13. Howden CV and Hunt RH: Relationship between gastric secretion and infection. Gut 28:96–107, 1987.

14. Mojaverian P, et al.: Estimation of gastric residence time of the Heidelberg capsule in humans. Gastroenterol 89:392–7, 1985.

15. Wright J: A proposal for standardized challenge testing of gastric acid secretory capacity using the Heidelberg capsule radiotelemetry system. J John Bastyr Col Nat Med 1:2:3–11, 1979.

16. Rubinstein E, et al.: Antibacterial activity of the pancreatic fluid. Gastroenterol 88:927–32, 1985.

17. Sarker SA and Gyr R: Non-immunological defense mechanisms of the gut. Gut 33:1331–7, 1990.

18. Oelgoetz AW, et al.: The treatment of food allergy and indigestion of pancreatic origin with pancreatic enzymes. Am J Dig Dis Nutr 2:422–6, 1935.

Chapter 4: Dietary Factors

1. Truss O: The Missing Diagnosis. POB 26508, Birmingham, AL, 1983.

2. Crook WG: The Yeast Connection, 2nd ed. Professional Books, Jackson, TN, 1984.

3. Kroker GF: Chronic candidiasis and allergy. In: Brostoff J and Challacombe SJ (eds): Food Allergy and Intolerance. WB Saunders, Philadelphia, 1987, pp. 850–72.

4. Crook WG: The Yeast Connection and the Woman. Professional Books, Jackson, TN, 1995.

5. Wright JV: Healing with Nutrition. Rodale, Emmaus, PA, 1984.

6. Dickey LD: Clinical Ecology, Thomas, Springfield, IL, 1974.

7. Taub EL: Food Allergy and the Allergic Patient. Thomas, Springfield, IL 1978.

8. Brostoff J and Challacombe SJ (eds): Food Allergy and Intolerance. WB Saunders, Philadelphia, 1987.

9. McGovern JJ: Correlation of clinical food allergy symptoms with serial pharmacological and immunological changes in the patient's plasma. Ann Allergy 44:57, 1980.

10. Ader R (ed): Psychoimmunology. Academic Press, New York, 1981.

11. Dockhorn RJ and Smith TC. Use of a chemically defined hypoallergenic diet in the management of patients with suspected food allergy. Ann Allergy 47:264–66, 1981.

12. Rowe AH and Rowe A: Food Allergy. Its Manifestations and Control and the Elimination Diets. CC Thomas, Springfield, IL, 1972.

13. Metcalfe D: Food hypersensitivity. J All Clin Imm 73:749–61, 1984.

14. Coca AF: Art of investigating pulse diet record in familial nonreagenic food allergy. Ann Allergy 2:1, 1944.

15. Rinkel HJ, Randolph T, and Zeller M: Food Allergy. CC Thomas, Springfield, IL, 1951.

16. Rinkel HJ: Food allergy IV: The function and clinical application of the rotary diversified diet. J Pediat 32:266, 1948.

17. National Research Council: Diet and Health. Implications for Reducing Chronic Disease Risk. National Academy Press, Washington, D.C., 1989.

18. Cheng KK, et al.: Pickled vegetables in the aetiology of oesophageal cancer in Hong Kong Chinese. Lancet 339:1314–8, 1992.

19. Anderson JW and Gustafson NJ: Dietary fiber in disease prevention and treatment. Compr Ther 13:43–53, 1987.

20. Fraser GE, Sabate J, Beeson WL, and Strahan TM: A possible protective effect of nut consumption on risk of coronary heart disease. Arch Intern Med 152:1416–24, 1992.

Chapter 5: Nutritional Supplementation

1. National Research Council: Recommended Dietary Allowances, 10th ed.. National Academy Press, Washington, D.C., 1989.

2. Murray MT: Encyclopedia of Nutritional Supplements. Prima, Rocklin, CA, 1996.

3. Galland L: Nutrition and candidiasis. J Orthomol Psych 15:50–60, 1985.

4. Samaranayake LP: Nutritional factors and oral candidosis. J Oral Pathol 15:61–5, 1986.

Chapter 6: Enhancing Immunity

1. Fridkin M and Najjar VA: Tuftsin: Its chemistry, biology, and clinical potential. Crit Rev Biochem Mol Biol 24:1–40, 1989.

2. Rastogi A, et al.: Augmentation of human natural killer cells by splenopentin analogs. FEBS Lett 317:93–5, 1993.

3. Minter MM: Agranulocytic angina: Treatment of a case with fetal calf spleen. Texas State J Med 2:338–43, 1933.

4. Gray GA: The treatment of agranulocytic angina with fetal calf spleen. Texas State J Med 29:366–9, 1933.

5. Iwata K: Toxins produced by *Candida albicans.* Contr Microbiol Immunol 4:77–85, 1977.

6. Axelson NH: Analysis of human *Candida precipitins* by quantitative immunoelectrophoresis. Scand J Immunol 5:177–90, 1976.

7. Cousins N: Anatomy of an Illness. Bantam Books, New York, 1979.

8. Dillon KM and Minchoff B: Positive emotional states and enhancement of the immune system. Intern J Psych Med 15:13–7, 1986.

9. Martin RA and Dobbin JP: Sense of humor, hassles, and immunoglobulin A: Evidence for a stress-moderating effect of humor. Int J Psych Med 18:93–105, 1988.

10. Irwin M, et al.: Reduction of immune function in life stress and depression. Biol Psych 27:22–30, 1990.

11. O'Leary A: Stress, emotion, and human immune function. Psychol Bull 108:363–82, 1990.

12. Kiecolt-Glaser JK and Glaser R: Psychoneuroimmunology: Can psychological interventions modulate immunity? J Consult Clin Psychol 60:569–75, 1992.

13. Moldofsky H, et al.: The relationship of interleukin-1 and immune functions to sleep in humans. Psychosomat Med 48:309–18, 1986.

14. Kusaka Y, Kondou H, and Morimoto K: Healthy lifestyles are associated with higher natural killer cell activity. Prev Med 21:602–15, 1992.

15. Nekachi K and Imai K: Environmental and physiological influences on human natural killer cell activity in relation to good health practices. Jap J Cancer Res 83:789–805, 1992.

16. National Research Council: Diet and Health: Implications for Reducing Chronic Disease Risk. National Academy Press, Washington, D.C., 1989.

17. Galland L: Nutrition and candidiasis. J OrthomolPsych 15:50–60, 1985.

18. Samaranayake LP: Nutritional factors and oral candidosis. J Oral Pathol 15:61–5, 1986.

19. Palmblad J, Hallberg D, and Rossner S: Obesity, plasma lipids and polymorphonuclear (PMN) granulocyte functions. Scand J Heamatol 19:293–303, 1977.

20. Sanchez A, et al.: Role of sugars in human neutrophilic phagocytosis. Am J Clin Nutr 26:1180–4, 1973.

21. Ringsdorf W, Cheraskin E, and Ramsay R: Sucrose, neutrophil phagocytosis and resistance to disease. Dent Surv 52:46–8, 1976.

22. Bernstein J, et al.: Depression of lymphocyte transformation following oral glucose ingestion. Am J Clin Nutr 30:613, 1977.

23. Brown MB (ed): Present Knowledge in Nutrition, 6th ed. Nutrition Foundation, Washington, DC, 1990.

24. Beisel WR: Single nutrients and immunity. Am J Clin Nutr 35:S417–68, 1982.

25. Alexander M, Newmark H, and Miller R: Oral beta-carotene can increase the number of OKT4+ cells in human blood. Immunol Letters 9:221–4, 1985.

26. Dardenne M, et al.: Contribution of zinc and other metals to the biological activity of the serum thymic factor. Proc Natl Acad Sci 79:5370–3, 1982.

27. Bogden JD, et al.: Zinc and immunocompetence in the elderly: Baseline data on zinc nutriture and immunity in unsupplemented subjects. Am J Clin Nutr 46:101–9, 1987.

28. Edman J, Sobel JD, and Taylor ML: Zinc status in women with recurrent vulvovaginal candidiasis. Am J Obstet Gynecol 155:1082–5, 1986.

29. Cazzola P, Mazzanti P, and Bossi G: In vivo modulating effect of a calf thymus acid lysate on human T lymphocyte subsets

and CD4+/CD8+ ratio in the course of different diseases. Curr Ther Res 42:1011–7, 1987.

30. Kouttab NM, Prada M, and Cazzola P: Thymomodulin: Biological properties and clinical applications. Medical Oncol and Tumor Pharmacother 6:5–9, 1989.

Chapter 7: Promoting Detoxification

1. Regenstein L: America the Poisoned. Acropolis, Washington, DC, 1982.

2. Rutter M and Russell-Jones R (eds): Lead versus Health: Sources and Effects of Low Level Lead Exposure. John Wiley, New York, 1983.

3. Klein A, et al.: The effect of nonviral liver damage on the T-lymphocyte helper/suppressor ratio. Clin Immunol Immunopathol 46:214–20, 1988.

4. Abe F, Nagata S, and Hotchi M: Experimental candidiasis in liver injury. Mycopathologica 100:37–42, 1987.

5. Flora SJS, Singh S, and Tandon SK: Prevention of lead intoxication by vitamin B complex. Z Ges Hyg 30:409–11, 1984.

6. Shakman RA: Nutritional influences on the toxicity of environmental pollutants: A review. Arch Env Health 28:105–33, 1974.

7. Flora SJS, et al.: Protective role of trace metals in lead intoxication. Toxicol Letters 13:51–6, 1982.

8. Barak AJ, et al.: Dietary betaine promotes generation of hepatic S-adenosylmethionine and protects the liver from ethanol-induced fatty infiltration. Alcohol Clin Exp Res 17:552–5, 1993.

9. Zeisel SH, et al.: Choline, an essential nutrient for humans. FASEB J 5:2093–8, 1991.

10 Baker DH and Czarnecki-Maulden GL: Pharmacolic role of cysteine in ameliorating or exacerbating mineral toxicities. J Nutr 117:1003–10, 1987.

11. Hikino H, et al.: Antihepatotoxic actions of flavonolignans from *Silybum marianum* fruits. Planta Med 50:248–50, 1984.

12. Vogel G, et al.: Studies on pharmacodynamics, site and mechanism of action of silymarin, the antihepatotoxic principle from *Silybum marianum (L.) Gaert.* Arzneim.-Forsch 25:179–85, 1975.

13. Wagner H: Antihepatotoxic flavonoids. In: Plant Flavonoids in Biology and Medicine: Biochemical, Pharmacological, and Structure-Activity Relationships. Cody V, Middleton E, and Harbourne JB (ed). Alan R. Liss, New York, 1986, pp. 545–58.

14. Valenzuela A, et al.: Selectivity of silymarin on the increase of the glutathione content in different tissues of the rat. Planta Med 55:420–2, 1989.

15. Sarre H: Experience in the treatment of chronic hepatopathies with silymarin. Arzneim.-Forsch 21:1209–12, 1971.

16. Canini F, et al.: Use of silymarin in the treatment of alcoholic hepatic steatosis. Clin Ter 114:307–14, 1985.

17. Salmi HA and Sarna S: Effect of silymarin on chemical, functional, and morphological alteration of the liver: A double-blind controlled study. Scand J Gastroenterol 17:417–21, 1982.

18. Boari C, et al.: Occupational toxic liver diseases: Therapeutic effects of silymarin. Min Med 72:2679–88, 1985.

19. Ferenci P, et al.: Randomized controlled trial of silymarin treatment in patients with cirrhosis of the liver. J Hepatol 9:105–13, 1989.

20. Imamura M and Tung T: A trial of fasting cure for PCB poisoned patients in Taiwan. Am J Ind Med 5:147–53, 1984.

Chapter 8: Probiotics

1. Metchnikoff E: The Prolongation of Life. Arna Press, New York, 1908 (1977 reprint).

2. Hentges DJ: Human intestinal microflora. In: Health and Disease. Hentges, DJ (ed.). Academic Press, New York, 1983.

3. Shahani KM and Ayebo AD: Role of dietary lactobacilli in gastrointestinal microecology. Am J Clin Nutr 33:2448–57, 1980.

4. Shahani KM and Friend BA: Nutritional and therapeutic aspects of lactobacilli. J Appl Nutr 36:125–52, 1984.

5. Hughes VL and Hillier SL: Microbiologic characteristics of lactobacillus products used for colonization of the vagina. Obstet Gynecol 75:244–8, 1990.

6. Mitsuoka T: Intestinal flora and host. Asian Med J 31:400–9, 1988.

7. Barefoot SF, and Klaenhammer TR: Detection and activity of lacticin B, a bacteriocin produced by *Lactobacillus acidophilus.* Appl Environ Microbiol 45:1808–15, 1983.

8. Klaenhammer TR: Microbiological considerations in the selection of preparations of lactobacillus strains for use in dietary adjuncts. J Dairy Sci 65:1339–49, 1982.

9. Klaenhammer TR: Bacteriocins of lactic acid bacteria. Biochemie 70:337–49, 1988.

10. Upreti GC and Hinsdill RD: Isolation and characterization of a bacteriocin from a homofermentative Lactobacillus. Antimicrob Agents Chemother 4:487–94, 1973.

11. Upreti GC and Hinsdill RD: Production and mode of action of lactocin 27: Bacteriocin from a homofermentative Lactobacillus. Antimicrob Agents Chemother 7:139–45, 1975.

12. DeKlerk HC: Bacteriocinogency in Lactobacillus fermenti. Nature 214:609, 1967.

13. DeKlerk HC and Smit JA: Properties of a Lactobacillus fermenti bacteriocin. J Gen Microbiol 48:309–16, 1967.

14. Friend BA and Shahani KM: Nutritional and therapeutic aspects of lactobacilli. J Appl Nutr 36:125–52, 1984.

15. Shahani KM, Vakil JR, and Kilara A: Natural antibiotic activity of *Lactobacillus acidophilus* and *bulgaricus:* II. Isolation of acidophilin from *L. acidophilus.* Cult Dairy Prod J 12:8, 1977.

16. Shahani KM, Vakil JR, and Kilara A: Natural antibiotic activity of *Lactobacillus acidophilus* and *Lactobacillus bulgaricus.* Cult Dairy Prod J 11:14–7, 1976.

17. Dahiya RS and Speck ML: Hydrogen peroxide formation by lactobacilli and its effect on *Staphylococcus aureus.* J Dairy Sci 51:1568, 1968.

18. Price RJ and Lee JS: Inhibition of pseudomonas species by hydrogen-peroxide producing lactobacilli. J Milk Food Technol 33:13, 1970.

19. Vesely R, Negri R, Bianchi-Salvadori B, et al.: Influence of a diet addition with yogurt on the mouse immune system. EOS J Immunol Immunopharmacol 5:30–5, 1985.

20. Vincent JG, Veonett RC, and Riley RG: Antibacterial activities associated with *Lactobacillus acidophilus.* J Bacteriol 78:477, 1959.

21. Perdigon G, N de Macias ME, Alvarez S, et al.: Enhancement of immune response in mice fed with *Streptococcus thermophilus* and *Lactobacillus acidophilus.* J Dairy Sci 70:919–26, 1987.

22. Weir D and Blackwell C: Interaction of bacteria with the immune system. J Clin Lab Immunol 10:1–12, 1983.

23. Perdigon G, N de Macias ME, Alvarez S, et al.: Systemic augmentation of the immune response in mice by feeding fermented milks with *Lactobacillus casei* and *Lactobacillus acidophilus.* Immunol 63:17–23, 1988.

24. Perdigon G, et al.: Symposium: Probiotic bacteria for humans: Clinical systems for evaluation of effectiveness. Immune system stimulation by probiotics. J Dairy Sci 78:1597–1606, 1995.

25. Clements ML, Levine MM, Black RE, et al.: Lactobacillus prophylaxis for diarrhea due to enterotoxinogenic *Escherichia coli.* Antimicrob Agents Chemotherap 20:104–8, 1981.

26. Dios Pozo-Olano JD, Warram JH, Gomez RG, and Cavazos MG: Effect of a lactobacilli preparation on traveler's diarrhea: A randomized, double-blind clinical trial. Gastroenterol 74:829–30, 1978.

27. Thompson GE: Control of intestinal flora in animals and humans: Implications for toxicology and health. J Environ Path Toxicol 1:113–23, 1977.

28. Clements ML, Levine MM, and Ristaino PA: Exogenous lactobacilli fed to man: Their fate and ability to prevent diarrheal disease. Prog Food Nutr Sci 7:29–37, 1983.

29. Zoppi G, Deganello A, Benoni G, and Saccomani F: Oral bacteriotherapy in clinical practice: I. The use of different preparations in infants treated with antibiotics. Eur J Ped 139:18–21, 1982.

30. Gotz VP, Romankiewics JA, Moss J, and Murray HW: Prophylaxis against ampicillin-induced diarrhea with a lactobacillus preparation. Am J Hosp Pharm 36:754–7, 1979.

31. Zoppi G, Balsamo V, Deganello A, et al.: Oral bacteriotherapy in clinical practice. I. The use of different preparations in the treatment of acute diarrhea. Eur J Ped 139:22–4, 1982.

32. Collins EB and Hardt P: Inhibition of *Candida albicans* by *Lactobacillus acidophilus.* J Dairy Sci 63:830–2, 1980.

33. Butler C and Beakley JW: Bacterial flora in the vagina. Am J Obstet Gynecol 79:432, 1960.

34. Lock FR, Yow MD, Griffith MI, and Stout M: Bacteriology of the vagina in 75 normal young adults. Surg Gyn Obs 87:410, 1948.

35. Rogosa M and Sharp ME: Species differentiation of human vaginal lactobacilli. J Gen Microbiol 23:197, 1960.

36. Wylie JG and Henderson A: Identity of glycogen-fermenting ability of lactobacilli isolated from the vagina of pregnant women. J Med Microbiol 2:363, 1969.

37. Huppert M, Cazin J, and Smith H: Pathogenesis of *C. albicans* infections following antibiotic therapy. J Bacterio 70:440–7, 1955.

38. Neri A, Sabah G, and Samra Z: Bacterial vaginosis in pregnancy treated with yoghurt. Acta Obstet Gynecol 72:17–19, 1993.

39. Reid G, Bruce AW, and Taylor M: Influence of three-day antimicrobial therapy and lactobacillus vaginal suppositories on recurrence of urinary tract infections. Clin Ther 14:11–6, 1992.

40. Tomomatsu H: Health effects of oligosaccharides. Food Technol October:61–5, 1994.

41. Gibson GR, et al.: Selective stimulation of bifidobacteria in the human colon by oligofructose and inulin. Gastroenterol 108:975–82, 1995.

Chapter 9: Natural and Prescription Anti-Yeast Agents

1. Keeney EL: Sodium caprylate: A new and effective treatment of moniliasis of the skin and mucous membrane. Bull Johns Hopkins Hosp 78:333–9, 1946.

2. Neuhauser I and Gustus EL: Successful treatment of intestinal moniliasis with fatty acid resin complex. Arch Intern Med 93:53–60, 1954.

3. Scwhabe AD, Bennett LR, and Bowman LP: Octanoic acid absorption and oxidation in humans. J Applied Physiol 19:335–7, 1964.

4. Hahn FE and Ciak J: Berberine. Antibiotics 3:577–88, 1976.

5. Amin AH, Subbaiah TV, and Abbasi KM: Berberine sulfate: Antimicrobial activity, bioassay, and mode of action. Can J Microbiol 15:1067–76, 1969.

6. Johnson CC, Johnson G, and Poe CF: Toxicity of alkaloids to certain bacteria. Acta Pharmacol Toxicol 8:71–8, 1952.

7. Kaneda, Y et al.: In vitro effects of berberine sulfate on the growth of *Entamoeba histolytica, Giardia lamblia,* and *Tricomonas vaginalis.* Annals Trop Med Parasitol 85:417–25, 1991.

8. Subbaiah TV and Amin AH: Effect of berberine sulfate on *Entamoeba histolytica.* Nature 215:527–8, 1967.

9. Ghosh AK: Effect of berberine chloride on *Leishmania donovani.* Ind J Med Res 78:407–16, 1983.

10. Majahan VM, Sharma A, and Rattan A: Antimycotic activity of berberine sulphate: An alkaloid from an Indian medicinal herb. Sabouraudia 20:79–81, 1982.

11. Gupta S: Use of berberine in the treatment of giardiasis. Am J Dis Child 129:866, 1975.

12. Bhakat MP, et al.: Therapeutic trial of berberine sulphate in non-specific gastroenteritis. Ind Med J 68:19–23, 1974.

13. Kamat SA: Clinical trial with berberine hydrochloride for the control of diarrhoea in acute gastroenteritis. J Assoc Physicians India 15:525–9, 1967.

14. Desai AB, Shah KM, and Shah DM: Berberine in the treatment of diarrhoea. Ind Pediatr 8:462–5, 1971.

15. Sharma R, Joshi CK, and Goyal RK: Berberine tannate in acute diarrhea. Ind Pediatr 7:496–501, 1970.

16. Choudry VP, Sabir M, and Bhide VN: Berberine in giardiasis. Ind Pediatr 9:143–6, 1972.

17. Kamat SA: Clinical trial with berberine hydrochloride for the control of diarrhoea in acute gastroenteritis. J Assoc Physicians India 15:525–9, 1967.

18. Gupte S: Use of berberine in treatment of giardiasis. Am J Dis Child 129:866, 1975.

19. Rabbani GH, et al.: Randomized controlled trial of berberine sulfate therapy for diarrhea due to enterotoxigenic *Escherichia coli* and *Vibrio cholerae.* J Infect Dis 155:979–84, 1987.

20. Hladon B: Toxicity of berberine sulfate. Acta Pol Pharm 32:113–20, 1975.

21. Moore GS and Atkins RD: The fungicidal and fungistatic effects of an aqueous garlic extract on medically important yeast-like fungi. Mycologia 69:341–8, 1977.

22. Sandhu DK, Warraich MK, and Singh S: Sensitivity of yeasts isolated from cases of vaginitis to aqueous extracts of garlic. Mykosen 23:691–8, 1980.

23. Prasad G and Sharma VD: Efficacy of garlic (*Allium sativum*) treatment against experimental candidiasis in chicks. Br Vet J 136:448–51, 1980.

24. Stiles JC, et al.: The inhibition of *Candida albicans* by oregano. J Appl Nutr 47:96–102, 1995.

Chapter 10: Special Concerns for Women

1. Heidrich F, et al.: Clothing factors and vaginitis. J Fam Prac 19:491–4, 1984.
2. Kudelco N: Allergy in chronic monilial vaginitis. Ann Allergy 29:266–7, 1971.
3. Shook D: A clinical study of a povidone iodine regimen for resistant vaginitis. Curr Ther Res 5:256–63, 1963.
4. Maneksha S: Comparison of povidone iodine (Betadine) vaginal pessaries and lactic acid pessaries in the treatment of vaginitis. J Int Med Res 2:236–9, 1974.
5. Reeve P: The inactivation of *Chlamydia trachomatis* by povidone iodine. J Antimicrob Chemo 2:77–80, 1976.
6. Ratzen J: Monilial and trichomonal vaginitis: Topical treatment with povidone iodine treatments. Cal Med 110:24–7, 1969.
7. Mayhew S: Vaginitis: A study of the efficacy of povidone iodine in unselected cases. J Int Med Res 9:157–9, 1981.
8. Swate T and Weed J: Boric acid treatment of vulvovaginal candidiasis. Ob Gyn 43:894–5, 1974.
9. Keller Van Slyke K: Treatment of vulvovaginal candidiasis with boric acid powder. Am J Ob Gyn 141:145–8, 1981.
10. Meeker CI: Candidiasis: An obstinate problem. Med Times 106:26–32, 1978.
11. Solomons CC, Melmed MH, and Heitler SM: Calcium citrate for vulvar vestibulitis. J Reprod Med 36:879–82, 1991.
12. Hornig DH, Moser U, and Glatthaar BE: Ascorbic Acid. In: Modern Nutrition in Health and Disease, 7th ed. Shils ME and Young VR (eds). Lea and Febiger, Philadelphia, 1988, pp. 417–35.
13. Editorial: Citrate for calcium nephrolithiasis. Lancet i:955, 1986.
14. Pak CYC and Fuller C: Idiopathic hypocitraturic calcium-oxalate nephrolithiasis successfully treated with potassium citrate. Ann Int Med 104:33–7, 1986.

Index

A

Achlorhydria, 36
Acidifying the urine, 23–24
Acne, 29–32
Alcohol, liver function and,
    104–105
Alkalinizing the urine, 23–24
Allergy to foods. *See* Food
    allergies
American Academy of Environ-
    mental Medicine, 9
American Association of Natur-
    opathic Physicians, 9
American College of
    Advancement in Medicine
    (ACAM), 9
American Holistic Medical
    Association, 9
*American Journal of Industrial
    Medicine,* 108
*American Journal of Natural
    Medicine, The,* v
Amylases (pancreatic enzymes),
    38–41
Anatomy of an Illness, 90

Angelica, for PMS, 144
Animal foods
    in candida control diet, 72
    milk and dairy products, 45, 72
    taxonomic list of animals, 60
*Annals of the Rheumatic
    Diseases,* 13
Antibiotics, 17–34
    for acne, 30, 31–32
    for bladder infections, 21
    candida overgrowth and,
        17–18
    dependence upon, 17, 18–19,
        27
    overuse of, 17
    post-antibiotic therapy, 18,
        118–119
    proper use of, 17–18
    resistance to, 33
    risks from using, 21, 27, 30,
        32–34
    for upper respiratory tract
        infections, 26–27
Antibodies
    cytotoxic reactions and, 50

Antibodies *(continued)*
  immediate hypersensitivity
    and, 49–50
  immune-complex mediated
    reactions and, 50–51
  measuring levels, 12
  in mucosal membrane, 51–52
  production of, 87
  types of, 49
Antibody Assay Laboratory, 12
Anti-fungal agents. *See* Anti-
    yeast agents
Antigens
  barrier against food anti-
    gens, 51–52
  cytotoxic reactions and, 50
  defined, 46, 49
  food allergies and, 49
  Herxheimer reaction, 123–124
  immediate hypersensitivity
    and, 49–50
  immune-complex mediated
    reactions and, 50–51
  measuring levels, 12
  secreted by *Candida albicans,*
    89
Antioxidants
  liver function and, 103, 105
  supplements, 77–80
  thymus function and, 96–97
  vegetables as sources, 64
  vitamins C and E, 78–80
Anti-ulcer drugs, 35–36
Anti-yeast agents, 123–130
  boric acid vs., 134–135
  Herxheimer reaction, 123–124
  natural, 124–127
  prescription, 127–129
Aqueous-phase antioxidants,
    78–79
Arctostaphylos uva ursi, 25
Attitude, immune function and,
    90–91
Azole drugs, 128–129

B
Bacteria. *See also* Probiotics
  antibiotic resistance, 33

bladder infections from, 20
  inhibited by *L. acidophilus,*
    118
  lactobacilli in human intes-
    tine, 115
  probiotics (friendly), 21,
    113–121
  small intestinal bacterial
    overgrowth, 13–14
Basophils, 46, 86
  mast cells, 46, 87–88
B cells, 87
Beans (legumes), 59, 68–69
Bearberry (uva ursi), 25
Berberine-containing plants, 25,
    125–126. *See also* Gold-
    enseal
Bernard, Claude, 18–19
Betaine (lipotropic agents),
    106–107
Bifidobacterium bifidum. See also
    Probiotics
  available forms, 114–116
  dosage issues, 120–121
  introduction in infants, 114
  post-antibiotic therapy,
    118–119
  in probiotics, 113
Black cohosh, 145
Bladder infections, 19–26
  acidifying or alkalinizing
    urine, 23–24
  antibiotics for, 21
  causes of, 20
  herbal medicines, 24–26
  increasing urine flow, 21–23
  natural approach to, 21–26
Blood tests for food allergy,
    56–57
B-lymphocytes, 85
Boric acid, 134–135
Bromelain, 28–29
Bronchitis. *See* Upper respira-
    tory tract infections

C
Calcium citrate, 139–140
Calcium oxalate, 138–139

Cancer
  grains and, 67
  pickled vegetables and, 65
Candida albicans
  Herxheimer reaction, 123–124
  natural anti-yeast agents,
    124–127
  prescription anti-yeast thera-
    pies, 127–129
  toxins and antigens secreted
    by, 89
Candida control diet, 63–74
  fats, 70–71
  fruits, 73–74
  grains, 67–68
  legumes (beans), 68–69
  meats, fish, and eggs, 72
  milk and dairy products, 72
  nuts and seeds, 69–70
  vegetables, 63–67
Candida cycle, 2, 4
Candidiasis. *See* Chronic
  candidiasis
Caprylic acid, 124
Carbohydrates. *See* Sugars
CDSA (comprehensive digestive
  stool analysis), 10–12
Cell-mediated immunity, 84
Chlamydia, 84
Choline (lipotropic agents),
  106–107
Chronic candidiasis
  candida cycle, 2, 4
  causes, 2, 3
  diagnosis, 8–12
  immune function and, 88–89
  liver damage and, 103
  overview, 1–2
  questionnaire, 3, 5–8
  related syndromes, 12–16
  step-by-step approach,
    147–149
  typical patient profile, 3
Cimetidine (Tagamet), 35
Cimicifuga racemosa, 145
Citrate salts
  for alkalinizing urine, 23–24
  for vulvodynia, 139–140
Complement fractions, 88

Complete protein, 68
Complex carbohydrates, 44–45
Comprehensive digestive stool
  analysis (CDSA), 10–12
Cooking vegetables, 64
Cousins, Norman, 90
Cranberries and cranberry juice,
  22–23
Crohn's disease, 33–34
Crook, William, 1, 137
Cycle of candida overgrowth, 2, 4
Cytotoxic reactions, 50

D
Dairy products, 45, 72
Degenerative diseases, diet and,
  64, 67, 73
Depression, immune function
  and, 90–91
Detoxification, 101–112
  diet and, 104
  fasting for, 108–111
  lifestyle and, 104–105
  liver and, 101–111
  liver detoxification profile,
    112
  nutritional supplements,
    105–108
  promoting elimination, 111
Diabetics, free radicals and, 64
Diagnosis. *See also* Symptoms;
    Tests
  comprehensive digestive
    stool analysis (CDSA),
    10–12
  of food allergies, 54–57
  of leaky gut syndrome, 15–16
  overview, 8–9
  questionnaire, 3, 5–8
  self-diagnosis, x
  of small intestinal bacterial
    overgrowth, 13–14
Diagnos-Techs, 10, 12, 112
Diet
  avoiding allergenic foods,
    57–58
  candida control diet, 63–74
  elimination diet, 54–56

Diet *(continued)*
    food families, 59–60
    immune function and, 94–96
    importance of, 74
    liver function and, 103, 104
    nutrient deficiency, 94–96
    for respiratory tract infec-
        tions, 28
    Rotary Diversified Diet, 58–63
    for vulvodynia treatment,
        138–139
Dietary factors. *See also* Food
        allergies
    food allergies, 45–63
    milk and dairy products, 45
    mold- and yeast-containing
        foods, 45
    nutrient deficiency, 94–96
    sugars, 43–45
Diflucan (fluconazole), 128–129
Digestive analysis (CDSA),
        10–12
Digestive secretions, 35–41
    hypochlorhydria, 35–38
    importance of, 35
    pancreatic enzymes, 38–41
Doctors. *See* Physicians
Dong quai, for PMS, 144
Drugs. *See* Antibiotics; Medica-
        tions
Dyspareunia, 136

E
E. coli, 20, 22–23
Eggs. *See* Animal foods
Elimination
    fasting, 108–111
    promoting, 111
Elimination diet, 54–55
ELISA (enzyme-linked
        immunosorbent assay)
        test, 56–57
Enteric-coated volatile oils, 127
Eosinophils, 86
Erythromycin, 30. *See also*
        Antibiotics
Escherichia coli, 20, 22–23

Essential fatty acids, 70–71,
        80–81
Exercise, liver function and, 104

F
Fasting
    before food-challenge test-
        ing, 54, 55–56
    caution concerning, 109
    for detoxification, 108–111
    three-day juice fast, 109–110
    tips, 110–111
Fats
    about, 70–71
    in candida control diet, 71
    essential fatty acids, 70–71,
        80–81
    obesity and, 95
Fatty acids, 70–71, 80–81
Fermented foods, 113–114
Fiber formulas, 111
Fibroids, uterine, 145
Fish. *See* Animal foods
Flaxseed oil, 80–81
Flora, intestinal. *See* Probiotics
Fluconazole (Diflucan), 128–129
Food allergies, 45–63
    avoiding allergenic foods,
        57–58
    causes, 48–51, 52–54
    cyclic vs. fixed, 46
    cytotoxic reactions, 50
    dealing with, 57–63
    described, 45–46
    diagnosis, 54–57
    immediate hypersensitivity,
        49–50
    immune-complex mediated
        reactions, 50–51
    immune system disorders
        and, 51–52
    nonimmunological mecha-
        nisms, 53–54
    prevalence of, 47
    Rotary Diversified Diet, 58–63
    symptom process, 48
    symptoms, 46–48

T-cell dependent reactions, 51
triggering factors, 46, 52–54
Food anaphylaxis. *See* Food
allergies
Food challenge, 54–56
Food families, 59–60
Food hypersensitivity. *See* Food
allergies
Food idiosyncrasy. *See* Food
allergies
Food intolerance. *See* Food
allergies
Food sensitivity. *See* Food
allergies
FOS (fructo-oligosaccharides),
120
"Free foods," 66–67
Free radicals, 64, 77
Friendly bacteria. *See* Pro-
biotics
Fructo-oligosaccharides (FOS),
120
Fruits, 60, 73–74

G
Garlic, 126
Gastric acid analysis, Heidel-
berg, 36
Gentian violet, 136
Germ theory, 18–19
Glutathione, 107
Glycyrrhiza glabra, for PMS, 144
Goldenseal
for bladder infections, 25–26
dosage, 26
other berberine-containing
plants, 25, 125–126
for respiratory tract infec-
tions, 28
Grains, 59, 67–68
Great Smokies Diagnostic Labo-
ratory, 10, 112

H
Happiness, immune function
and, 90–91

Heidelberg gastric acid analysis,
36
Herbal medicines
berberine-containing plants,
25, 125–126
for bladder infections, 24–26
enhancing immune function,
98–99
enteric-coated volatile oils, 127
garlic, 126
milk thistle (silymarin),
107–108
for PMS, 144–145
Herxheimer reaction, 123–124
Hormones, 84–85, 91
Hydrastis canadensis. See
Goldenseal
Hydrochloric acid
supplements, 36–38
test for, 36
Hypochlorhydria, 35–38
anti-ulcer drugs and, 35–36
defined, 36
diseases associated with, 37
Heidelberg gastric acid
analysis, 36
hydrochloric acid supple-
ments for, 36–38
symptoms, 37

I
Immediate hypersensitivity, 49–50
Immune-complex mediated
reactions, 50–51
Immune system, 83–99. *See also*
Antibodies; Food allergies
causes of depressed immune
function, 89, 90
depressed immune function
in chronic candidiasis,
88–89
diet and, 94–96
disorders and food allergies,
51–52
immune-mediated reactions
to food, 49–51
lifestyle and, 93–94

Immune system *(continued)*
  liver and immune function, 102
  lymph, lymphatic vessels, and lymph nodes, 85
  mood and attitude influence on, 90–91
  nutrient deficiency and, 94–96
  overview, 83–88
  plant-based medicines for, 98–99
  restoring immune function, 89–99
  sleep and, 92, 94
  special chemical factors, 88
  special tissue cells, 87–88
  spleen, 85–86
  stress and, 91–93
  thymus function, 84–85, 96–98
  white blood cells, 86–88
Immunodiagnostic Lab, 12
Infections
  bladder infections, 19–26
  small intestinal bacterial overgrowth, 13–14
  urinary tract infections, 22–23
  vaginal yeast infections, 131–136
Inheritance of food allergy, 48–49
Intercourse, painful, 136
Interferon, 88
Interleukin II, 88
Internal terrain, 18–19
Interstitial fluid, 85
Interstitium, 85
Intestines
  lactobacilli in, 115
  promoting healthy environment, 116–118
  small intestinal bacterial overgrowth, 13–14
Iodine, 134
Itroconazole (Sporanox), 128–129

K
Ketoconazole (Nizoral), 128–129
Kupffer cells, 102

L
Laboratories. *See also* Tests
  for blood tests for food allergy, 57
  for comprehensive digestive stool analysis (CDSA), 10–12
  for liver detoxification profile, 112
  for measuring antibody or antigen levels, 12
  for urinary oxalate measurement, 140
Lactobacilli. *See* Probiotics
Lactobacillus acidophilus. See also Probiotics
  anti-microbial activity, 117–118
  available forms, 114–116
  for bladder infections, 21
  DDS-1 "super-strain," 116
  dosage issues, 120–121
  historical perspective, 113–114
  introduction in infants, 114
  post-antibiotic therapy, 118–119
  in probiotics, 113
  for vaginal yeast infections, 119, 133–134
Lactulose, leaky gut diagnosis and, 15–16
Lancet, The, 27
Laughter, 90–91
Laxatives, 111
Leaky gut syndrome, 14–16
Legumes (beans), 59, 68–69
Licorice root, for PMS, 144
Lifestyle, 28, 93–94, 104–105
Lipases (pancreatic enzymes), 38–41
Lipid-phase antioxidants, 79

Lipotropic agents, 106–107
Liver
  damage, chronic candidiasis
    and, 103
  detoxification profile, 112
  diet and, 103, 104
  fasting and detoxification,
    108–111
  immune function and, 102
  importance of, 101–102
  lifestyle and, 104–105
  lipotropic agents for,
    106–107
  signs of impaired function,
    105–106
  silymarin for, 107–108
  supporting liver function,
    103–111
Low oxalate diet, 138–139
Lymph, 85
Lymphatic vessels, 85
Lymph nodes, 85

M
Macrophages, 85, 87
Mannitol, 15–16
Mast cells, 46, 87–88
Meats. *See* Animal foods
Medications. *See also* Anti-
    biotics; Herbal medicines
  anti-ulcer drugs, 35–36
  anti-yeast therapies, 127–129
  discontinuing, x
  nutritional supplements and, x
Medicines, herbal. *See* Herbal
    medicines
Meridian Valley Clinical Labora-
    tory, 10, 57, 112
Metabolic reaction to food. *See*
    Food allergies
Metchnikoff, Elie, 19, 114
Methionine (lipotropic agents),
    106–107
Milk and dairy products, 45, 72
Milk thistle (silymarin), 107–108
Minerals
  liver function support, 105

multiple vitamin and mineral
    supplement, 75–77
Recommended Dietary
    Allowances (RDAs), 76–77
recommended ranges for
    adults, 79
Missing Diagnosis, The, 1
Mold-containing foods, 45, 70
Monocytes, 87
Mood, immune function and,
    90–91
Multiple vitamin and mineral
    supplement, 75–77
Murray, Michael T.
  about, v–vi
  books by, xiii
Mustard poultice, 29
Mycotoxins, 89

N
National BioTech Laboratory,
    10, 12, 57, 112
Natural killer cells, 87
Natural medicines, scientific
    nature of, v–vi
Neutrophils, 86
Nizoral (ketoconazole), 128–129
NK (natural killer) cells, 87
Nutritional supplements, 75–81
  antioxidants, 77–80
  in comprehensive treatment
    plan, xi
  discussing with doctor, x–xi
  flaxseed oil, 80–81
  hydrochloric acid, 36–38
  lipotropic agents, 106–107
  liver function support,
    105–108
  medications and, x
  multiple vitamin and mineral
    supplement, 75–77
  pancreatic enzymes, 38–41
  Recommended Dietary
    Allowances (RDAs), 76–77
  recommended ranges for
    adults, 78, 79
  silymarin, 107–108

Nutritional supplements
     (continued)
   for upper respiratory tract
     infections, 28
Nuts and seeds
   in candida control diet, 69–70
   fats, about, 71–72
   taxonomic list of, 59–60
Nystatin, 127–128

O

Obesity and immune function,
     95
Oligoantigenic (elimination)
     diet, 54–55
Oxalate, 138–139

P

Painful intercourse, 136
Pancreatic enzymes, 38–41
Pasteur, Louis, 18–19
Patient profile, typical, 3
Pharmacological reaction to
     food. *See* Food allergies
Physicians
   discussing nutritional sup-
     plements with, x–xi
   finding knowledgeable physi-
     cians, 9
   for PMS treatment, 145
   professional organizations, 9
Pickled vegetables, 65
Plant-based medicines. *See*
     Herbal medicines
Plants, edible, taxonomic list of,
     59–60
PMS. *See* Premenstrual
     syndrome
Postural drainage, 29
Potassium citrate, 23–24
Poultice, mustard, 29
Predisposing factors, 2, 3
Premenstrual syndrome,
     142–145
   herbal support, 144–145

need for physician, 145
   symptoms, 143
   treatment, 143–144
Prescription medicines. *See*
     Medications
Probiotics, 113–121
   available forms, 114–116
   defined, 113
   dosage issues, 120–121
   fructo-oligosaccharides for
     promoting, 120
   historical perspective, 113–114
   post-antibiotic therapy,
     118–119
   principle uses, 116
   promoting healthy intestinal
     environment, 116–118
   for urinary tract infections,
     21, 119
   for vaginal yeast infections,
     119, 133–134
Profile of typical patient, 3
Prostaglandins, 70–71
Proteases (pancreatic enzymes),
     38–41
Protein, complete, 68
Pruritis vulvae, 136
Psyllium-containing laxatives,
     111

Q

Questionnaire, 3, 5–8

R

Radio-allergo-sorbent test
     (RAST), 56–57
Ranitidine (Zantac), 35
Recommended Dietary
     Allowances (RDAs), 76–77
Resistance to antibiotics, 33
Respiratory tract infections,
     26–29
Rinkel, Herbert J., 58
Rotary Diversified Diet, 58–63
   food families, 59–60

four-day rotation diet, 61–63
overview, 58–59

S

Saturated fats, 70–71
Sci-Con, 140, 141
Seeds. *See* Nuts and seeds
Self-diagnosis, x
Shahani, Khem M., 116
Signs. *See* Symptoms
Silymarin, 107–108
Sinusitis. *See* Upper respiratory
    tract infections
Skin tests for food allergy, 56
Sleep, immune function and,
    92, 94
Small intestinal bacterial over-
    growth, 13–14
Sodium citrate, 23–24
Solomons, Clive C., 137–138
Sore throat. *See* Upper respira-
    tory tract infections
Spleen, immune system func-
    tion, 85–86
Sporanox (itraconazole), 128–129
Stool analysis (CDSA), 10–12
Stress
    coping with, 92–93
    immune function and, 91–92
Sugars, 43–45
    food labels and, 44
    immune function and, 95–96
    refined sugar, 43, 44
    simple vs. complex, 44–45
Supplements. *See* Nutritional
    supplements
Symptoms. *See also* Diagnosis;
    Tests
    candida questionnaire, 3, 5–8
    of food allergies, 46–48
    of hypochlorhydria, 37
    of leaky gut syndrome, 15
    of liver functions impair-
        ment, 105–106
    of small intestinal bacterial
        overgrowth, 13

typical patient profile, 3
vaginal yeast infections, 133
of vulvodynia, 136

T

Tagamet (cimetidine), 35
Taxonomic list of foods, 59–60
T cells, 51, 84, 86
Terrain, internal, 18–19
Tests. *See also* Diagnosis;
    Symptoms
    antibody or antigen levels, 12
    comprehensive digestive
        stool analysis (CDSA),
        10–12
    for food allergies, 56–57
    Heidelberg gastric acid
        analysis, 36
    liver detoxification profile,
        112
    pancreatic function assess-
        ment, 39
    for small intestinal bacterial
        overgrowth, 13–14
    urinary oxalate levels, 140,
        141
Tetracycline, 30, 31–32. *See also*
    Antibiotics
Thymulus, 98
Thymus extracts, 28, 98
Thymus gland, 84–85, 96–98
Truss, Orion, 1

U

Unsaturated fats, 70–71
Upland cranberry (uva ursi), 25
Upper respiratory tract infec-
    tions, 26–29
Urinary tract infections, 22–23,
    119
Urine
    acidifying or alkalinizing,
        23–24
    bladder infections and, 20
    increasing flow, 21–23

Uterine fibroids, 145
Uva ursi, 25

V
Vaginal yeast infections,
    131–136
  increase in, 131–132
  predisposing factors, 132
  reintroducing friendly bacte-
    ria, 119, 133–134
  symptoms, 133
  treatment, 119, 133–136
Vasoactive amines, 13
Vegetables, 59–60, 63–67
Vitamin B$_6$, thymus function
    and, 97
Vitamin C
  as antioxidant, 78–80
  for respiratory tract infec-
    tions, 28
  thymus function and, 97
Vitamin E, as antioxidant, 78–80
Vitamins
  liver function support, 105
  multiple vitamin and mineral
    supplement, 75–77
  Recommended Dietary
    Allowances (RDAs), 76–77
  recommended ranges for
    adults, 78
  thymus function and, 97
Volatile oils, enteric-coated, 127
Vulvar Pain Foundation, 137
Vulvodynia, 136–142
  case history, 140, 142
  symptoms, 136
  treatment, 138–140, 141, 142

W
Weight loss, "free foods" for,
    66–67
White blood cells
  immune system function,
    86–88
  Kupffer cells, 102
  production of, 85
  special tissue cells, 87–88
  types of, 86–87
Williams, Roger, 75
Women's concerns
  premenstrual syndrome,
    142–145
  urinary tract infections,
    22–23, 119
  vaginal yeast infections, 21,
    119, 131–136
  vulvodynia, 136–142

Y
*Yeast Connection and the
    Woman, The,* 137
Yeast Connection, The, 1
Yeast-containing foods, 45
Yeast inhibition by *L. aci-
    dophilus,* 118
Yeast syndrome. *See* Chronic
    candidiasis
Yogurt, friendly bacteria in, 115

Z
Zantac (ranitidine), 35
Zinc
  for acne, tetracycline vs., 31–32
  thymus function and, 97–98

Complete Candida Yeast Guidebook

*Everything You Need to Know About
Prevention, Treatment, and Diet*

Jeanne Marie Martin
with Zoltan Rona, M.D.

U.S. $18.95
Can. $25.95
ISBN 0-7615-0167-3
paperback / 456 pages

Proper diet is crucial in controlling the headaches, weight and digestive problems, and other complications of candida yeast syndrome. *Complete Candida Yeast Guidebook* will help you manage your yeast levels with complete diet plans, menus, and more than 200 delicious, nutritious recipes. Most are dairy-free and prepared without meat.

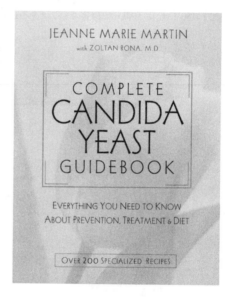

Written by a nutrition and natural foods expert with the assistance of a holistic medical doctor, this comprehensive resource also reviews the best treatments including natural remedies, prescription drugs, and lifestyle changes. You'll find simple diagnostic tests and encouraging case histories illustrating how others have overcome candida yeast syndrome.

GETTING WELL NATURALLY SERIES

Michael T. Murray, N.D.

In the highly successful GETTING WELL NATURALLY series, natural medicine researcher Dr. Michael T. Murray shares his extensive knowledge of herbs, exercise, and other natural healing methods with health-conscious readers. Dr. Murray's popular books help you understand and control chronic health problems and promote whole-body, physical, and emotional wellness. Each volume in the series provides natural programs, specific courses of treatment, dietary guidelines, and the latest information on a wide range of conditions.

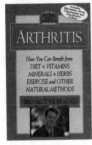

Arthritis
ISBN 1-55958-491-2
paperback / 176 pages
U.S. $11.00 / Can. $14.95

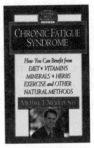

Chronic Fatigue Syndrome
ISBN 1-55958-490-4
paperback / 208 pages
U.S. $11.00 / Can. $14.95

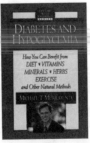

Diabetes & Hypoglycemia
ISBN 1-55958-426-2
paperback / 176 pages
U.S. $11.00 / Can. $16.00

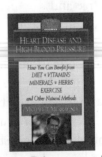

Heart Disease and High Blood Pressure
ISBN 0-7615-0658-6
paperback / 192 pages
U.S. $11.00 / Can. $16.00